613.25 DIE

The Diet advisor

Jasper County Public Library System

Overdue notices are a courtesy of
the library system.
Failure to receive an overdue notice
does not absolve the borrower of the
obligation to return materials on time.

TheDietAdvisor

health
magazine

TheDietAdvisor

The Complete Guide to Choosing the Right Diet for You

TIME
LIFE
BOOKS

TIME LIFE BOOKS • ALEXANDRIA, VIRGINIA

health
magazine

TIME INC HEALTH
Editor-in-Chief, *Health* magazine: Barbara Paulsen
Vice President/Publisher, *Health* magazine: Mary E. Morgan
Chief Operating Officer: Martha A. Lorini

The Diet Advisor
Food and Nutrition Editor, *Health* magazine:
Sheridan Warrick
Editor-in-Chief, Time Inc Health Custom Publishing:
John Poppy
Executive Editor, Time Inc Health Custom Publishing:
Eric Olsen

Time-Life Books is a division of Time Life Inc.
Time-Life is a trademark of Time Warner Inc.
and affiliated companies.

TIME LIFE INC.
CHAIRMAN AND CHIEF EXECUTIVE OFFICER: Jim Nelson
PRESIDENT AND CHIEF OPERATING OFFICER: Steven Janas
SENIOR EXECUTIVE VICE PRESIDENT AND CHIEF OPERATIONS
OFFICER: Mary Davis Holt
SENIOR VICE PRESIDENT AND CHIEF FINANCIAL OFFICER:
Christopher Hearing

TIME-LIFE BOOKS
PRESIDENT: Larry Jellen
SENIOR VICE PRESIDENT, NEW MARKETS: Bridget Boel
VICE PRESIDENT, HOME AND HEARTH MARKETS:
Nicholas M. DiMarco
VICE PRESIDENT, CONTENT DEVELOPMENT: Jennifer L. Pearce

TIME-LIFE TRADE PUBLISHING
VICE PRESIDENT AND PUBLISHER: Neil S. Levin
SENIOR SALES DIRECTOR: Richard J. Vreeland
DIRECTOR, MARKETING AND PUBLICITY: Inger Forland
DIRECTOR OF TRADE SALES: Dana Hobson
DIRECTOR OF CUSTOM PUBLISHING: John Lalor
DIRECTOR OF RIGHTS AND LICENSING: Olga Vezeris

THE DIET ADVISOR
DIRECTOR OF NEW PRODUCT DEVELOPMENT: Carolyn M. Clark
EXECUTIVE EDITOR: Robert Somerville
DIRECTOR OF DESIGN: Kate L. McConnell
TECHNICAL SPECIALIST: Monika Lynde
PAGE MAKEUP SPECIALIST: Jennifer Gearhart
PRODUCTION MANAGER: Vanessa Hunnibell
QUALITY ASSURANCE: Jim King and Stacy L. Eddy

Design: Studio A, Alexandria, Virginia

Consultant: Christine Ryan Spengler R.D.

Special Contributors: Constance Buchanan,
Teresa Graham, Rose Grant, Jane Harvey,
Susan Perry, Terrell Smith, Marilyn Terrell

Printed in U.S.A.
10 9 8 7 6 5 4 3 2 1

School and library distribution by Time-Life Education,
P.O. Box 85026, Richmond, Virginia 23285-5026.

CIP data available upon application:
Time-Life Books
2000 Duke Street
Alexandria, VA 22314

Books produced by Time-Life Trade Publishing are available
at a special bulk discount for promotional and premium use.
Custom adaptations can also be created to meet your specific marketing goals. Call 1-800-323-5255.

Visit the Time Life website at www.timelife.com

The information about health issues, diet, and exercise in
this book should be considered as a reference source only; it
is not intended to substitute for the advice of health professionals, including doctors, dieticians, and nutritionists. If
you plan to lose more than 15 or 20 pounds, have any health
problems, or take medication on a regular basis, you should
be evaluated by your doctor before beginning any weight-
loss or exercise program.

Contents

Foreword

Y ou *can* lose as many pounds as you want. You *can* keep them off. Those are the promises made by each and every one of the weight-control books we review in this special guide. We assembled it so you won't have to chew your way through one plan after another, searching for the one that fits.

We didn't choose the books at random, of course. If you just scan this month's bestseller list or stroll the aisles of any bookstore, you'll find these same volumes standing proud. As the editor of *Health* magazine, I've made sure that our award-winning writers and editors keep up with the very latest trends in weight loss and nutrition. We talk regularly with the authors of the best-selling diet books, we meet with successful dieters in their homes, and we consult top experts at their medical clinics and university labs. I can say without exaggerating that we know the ups and downs, the pluses and minuses of each of these weight-loss plans as well as anyone in the country.

So which one of them works best? The answer to that question shows up only when you plug yourself and your lifestyle into the equation. How soon do you expect to see results? How much free time do you have? Do you like to cook? Are you a self-starter or do you do prefer settings with plenty of group support? Have you tried to lose weight before and failed? Succeeded? Those are just some of the many questions you'll find yourself pondering as you dip into *The Diet Advisor* to find the plan that works best for you.

I encourage you to take your time in these pages, to be thoughtful and realistic—you owe it to yourself and to your future. Your sister and best friend may both have dropped a few dress sizes while following a low-carb diet, but that doesn't mean the same program will do as much for you. You're your own person. Your life is different.

One thing *is* common to all these plans: Whatever you're doing now, they require you to change it. All of them demand discipline, even devotion. They ask you to make tradeoffs and choices that may be hard—giving up favorite foods, for instance, or finding hours every week to exercise. Whatever a plan's particulars, we'll give you the details you need to make a wise choice right here in this guide. We'll even tell you when we think a diet may put your health at risk in return for a quick payoff. What we don't do is preach or wag our fingers. No guilt trips. You deserve to look good and feel good; you deserve the healthy body you want. We're committed to helping you get it.

Barbara Paulsen, editor-in-chief
Health magazine

A Guide to Good Dieting

Helping you choose the right diet for you—that's the promise of this book. And it's the motivation behind every one of the more than 20 reviews of weight-loss plans you'll find in *The Diet Advisor*. In each review, our goal is to give you a clear understanding of the diet—and an honest evaluation of its merits and demerits. But to really fulfill our promise, we need you to start here, with our "Guide to Good Dieting." Because whatever approach you choose, we feel strongly that it won't be right for you if it's not fundamentally healthy. The following pages, then, will give you a good grip on the basic principles of healthy eating—principles you can apply whether you're dieting or not. You'll get tips on making your chosen weight-loss plan work, as well as vital information on incorporating exercise into the plan. Finally, we'll give you practical advice on evaluating any diet—using the same criteria that helped us evaluate the diets in this book. If you take the time to read these pages first, you'll make even better use of the information in the reviews. And you'll be well on the way to successful, healthful dieting.

> Diet gurus preach their doctrines as if they were absolutes—and virtually every guru has a different doctrine.

Eating the Health-Wise Way

Trying to find the best way to slim down can be very confusing. Book upon book shouts one answer after another from the store shelves: elaborate low-fat or high-protein diets, body-sculpting plans almost calling for a masters in physiology, regimens of nutritional supplements so complex they'll turn your kitchen into a veritable pharmacy. Diet gurus preach their doctrines as if they were absolutes—and virtually every guru has a different doctrine.

Despite the impassioned pronouncements from these dietary pulpits, there really is no magic solution that works across the board. People put on pounds for many reasons: unhealthy diet, lack of exercise, emotional problems, even their genes. "No single dietary recommendation is right for everyone," says Ronald Krauss, a cholesterol researcher at Lawrence Berkeley National Laboratory in California. The old one-diet-fits-all mentality is fading, and that's good news for you. In your quest to shed pounds and keep them off, you can choose your own path, and chances are it will be more successful than any you might have tried in the past.

The paths are indeed many. A low-fat regimen may be the way to go for you. Or a slightly higher-fat one. You might want to graze throughout the day or eat three squares. Choose a Mediterranean diet or Chinese cuisine. Meticulously count calories or adopt a calorie-blind, overall healthy approach to eating. Perhaps you'll cherry-pick elements from several different diets and custom-design your own. But step one on any these paths needs to be an understanding of the basics of good nutrition.

Know Your Nutrients

To stay on a healthy course, your body requires a variety of nutrients: water, vitamins and minerals, carbohydrate, fat, and protein. These last three are the only nutrients that contain calories. A calorie is the amount of heat needed to raise the temperature of one liter of water by one degree centigrade. Calories are the energy that fuels your body.

The calorie-containing nutrient groups package their energy differently. Fat has nine calories per gram, while carbs and protein contain less than half that, at four calories per gram each. Figuring out the calorie content of a particular food from its gram weight isn't always a simple calculation, though, because the nutrient groups very often coexist in the same foods. Hamburger meat, for example, is both protein and fat, and regular milk contains protein, carb, and fat. Different foods, moreover, carry a different number of calories per volume. In foods that are primarily fatty, calories tend to be densely packed, meaning they deliver more calories for a given volume; in primarily protein foods they are less densely packed; and in primarily carbohydrate foods, calories are the least densely packed. For instance, you'd have to eat two heads of iceberg lettuce (a carb) to get 100 calories, and a mere tablespoon of butter to get the same number.

Carbohydrates

Carbohydrates are your body's number one fuel source. This class of carbon-based compounds includes sugars, starches, and cellulose. All carbohydrates must be broken down into glucose (blood sugar) to supply your body with energy. Simple sugars (fruit, honey) and double sugars (table sugar, milk) are digested quickly and give your body an energy surge. Complex carbohydrates (starchy and fibrous foods) are digested more slowly. The glucose that all these different carbohydrate types supply is your fuel, which you either use right away for energy, lodge in your muscle cells as potential energy (glycogen) or, if there's no room left in that inn, convert to fat and house in your fat cells.

Of all the body's food sources, complex carbohydrates supply the highest bulk value for the fewest calories. Many are dense in nutrients such as vitamins and minerals, and complex carbs also tend to pack lots of fiber, good news for dieters. You've heard it time and again: High-fiber, whole-grain carbs are far better for you than low-fiber carbs made from refined flour and sugar, the ingredients jammed into so many junk foods. Fiber passes out of your body and leaves behind very few calories. Moreover, it enhances and prolongs a feeling of fullness by slowing the absorption of foods. In delaying the absorption of glucose, fiber helps control blood sugar levels—a particularly important factor for people suffering from diabetes. Finally, soluble fiber—the sort that's found in oats, beans, and many types of produce—has been proven to help decrease LDL (low-density lipoprotein, the "bad" cholesterol) and triglycerides (fatty particles in the blood that can damage arteries), thereby reducing the risk of heart disease.

Carbohydrates are the main source of energy for your muscles when you exercise, and since exercise is crucial to healthy living, your body needs carbs.

Fat

The message seems loud and clear: Too much fat is gumming up our arteries, threatening our hearts—and making us fat. But the truth isn't quite so absolute. Fat is an essential component of healthy eating and performs a variety of vital functions. It enables your body to absorb certain minerals as well as the fat-soluble vitamins A, D, E, and K. It plays a role in hormone production and regulation, builds cell membranes, helps keep your skin lubricated, and plays a role in the healthy functioning of your immune system. It also keeps you warmer in winter and gives food flavor and texture.

Obviously, you cannot live on carbs and protein alone. But it is indeed true that you can have too much of a good thing. Fats teem with calories and tend to be low in nutrients. Most nutritional guidelines today recommend that people trying to lose weight derive no more than 30% of their calories from fat, and some professionals set that figure lower.

A word of caution about food labels: They can be very misleading when you're trying to determine how many calories you'll derive from fat in a given food. Labels on ground beef and milk, for example, list fat percentage by weight, not calories. So milk that is labeled as 2% fat—and touted as "low-fat"—does indeed have 2% fat by weight, but in terms of calories, it comes in at more than 35%. And "extra lean" ground beef, which might be labeled as 10% or even as low as 7% fat (the percentage by weight), actually derives as much as 65% of its calories from fat. It's all because fat is much denser in terms of calories than either carbs or protein.

Not all fats are equal. Saturated fat—completely saturated with hydrogen—tends to be solid at room temperature and is most commonly found in animal fat. Saturated fat abounds in butter, cheese, eggs, red meat, and coconut and palm oils. It's notorious for raising cholesterol and promoting heart disease.

There are several unsaturated fats—fats that are not saturated, or not completely saturated, with hydrogen. Polyunsaturated fats are prominent in corn, soybean, safflower, and sunflower oils. One type of polyunsaturated fat, omega-3, is found in

A word of caution about food labels: They can be very misleading.

most varieties of fish and is associated with a decreased risk of heart disease in certain people, probably because it can lower LDL cholesterol. But polyunsaturated fats are not all good news. In unadulterated form, polys have been shown to also lower high-density lipoprotein or HDL cholesterol, the "good" cholesterol that whisks LDL out of the bloodstream. Furthermore, of all fats polys, when heated, are most likely to form the DNA-damaging free radicals that are implicated in cancer.

Some polyunsaturated fats have hydrogen artificially added back to make them solid at room temperature. These are called partially hydrogenated, or trans, fats. They're found in crackers, commercial cookies, and most margarines. (The harder the margarine, the more it's hydrogenated, and the worse it is for you.) Trans fats can increase your chance of heart disease by lowering HDL and raising LDL. Moreover, when heated and reheated, as they are in fast-food restaurants that crank out chicken nuggets and French fries, trans fats form dangerous free radicals.

You can avoid a lot of these risks by sticking primarily with monounsaturated fats—resident in avocados and olive, canola, and peanut oil. Monounsaturated fats slightly lower LDL while slightly hiking HDL, thus helping prevent heart disease. Evidence suggests that olive oil may also play a role in preventing cancer. That's partly because olive oil is rich in plant-based antioxidants, which "mop up" the marauding free radicals that can damage DNA

If you have a choice, reach for the olive oil, not the margarine or butter. And watch out in particular for trans fats. They're likely be haunting those boxes on your grocery store shelf and those deep-fried meals in your fast-food restaurant.

Protein

Protein seems to have an enduring mythological status in the American diet. You are what you eat, the saying goes, and the popular notion is that dietary protein is imbued with miraculous properties that can make a person strong and lean. Not surprisingly, most Americans overconsume protein. Even without the myth, that wouldn't be hard to do. Protein exists in

If you have a choice, reach for the olive oil, not the margarine or butter.

almost everything you eat. You'll find it not just in meat, poultry, fish, dairy products, beans, and nuts—foods that are predominantly protein—but also in some fruits and vegetables.

Why do you need protein? It's made up of amino acids, the building blocks of all the tissue in your body—hair, skin, internal organs, and muscles. That doesn't mean protein is a magic muscle builder. You strengthen your muscles through exercise, not by overeating protein. But protein is important. In addition to building tissue, protein preserves the immune system, manufactures the enzymes and hormones that regulate bodily processes, and—in the absence of sufficient carbohydrates and fat—serves as fuel for the body. (Carbs, which are more easily digested, are the body's fuel of choice, followed by fat.)

If all protein foods were pure protein, weighing in at four calories per gram, overeating them wouldn't necessarily be bad. The problem is many protein foods come bundled with fat, at nine calories per gram, and worse yet, that fat tends to be saturated fat. Because of the fat connection, calories in predominantly protein foods are more densely packed than calories in predominantly carb foods, so you'll tend to eat more than you need for your basic fuel requirements if your diet is rich in protein foods.

Too much protein will just add to your waistline Yes, you need it, but remember, a little goes a long way.

Variety and Balance: The Food Guide Pyramid

You're probably familiar with it—the Food Guide Pyramid, that little picture that graces the side of your cereal box. In 1992 the U.S. Department of Agriculture issued this handy device to show at a glance the proportions of daily intake from each food group that should supply all the nutrients you need to maintain your health: six to 11 servings of grain foods, three to five servings of vegetables, two to four servings of fruit, two to three servings of milk, yogurt and/or cheese, two to three servings of meat, poultry, fish, beans, eggs, and/or nuts, and sparing use of fats and sweets.

> Protein isn't a magic muscle builder. You strengthen your muscles through exercise, not by overeating protein.

Who could eat all this and not turn into a blimp, you wonder. In fact, three-quarters of the servings come from the pyramid's lower tiers—the grains, veggies, and fruits. Almost all of these are low in calories and high in nutrients, if not processed or prepared with added fat (like French fries or potato chips). And compared to the average American serving in the home or most restaurants, the pyramid's servings are sparing: One serving equals half a cup of pasta, one slice of bread, one ounce of ready-to-eat cereal, a melon wedge, half a cup of cooked veggies. If you eat the minimum servings recommended and keep added fat and sweets to a minimum, the number of calories in your diet will be reasonable, and most likely low enough to promote weight loss.

The beauty of the pyramid? It's not prescriptive. You can eat what suits you, and as long as you adhere to its general principles of variety and balance, you'll know you're eating healthfully. Among other things, grains will provide you with B vitamins, fiber, and minerals such as iron. You'll get vitamins A and C, antioxidants, potassium, and fiber—to mention just a few—from veggies and fruits. Dairy foods will supply you with calcium and B vitamins. Poultry, fish, eggs, nuts, beans, and meat will meet various requirements including your need for protein, B vitamins, and iron.

Getting nutrients from all the groups may well be the best approach to healthy living, not to mention dieting and lifetime weight maintenance. "Food-specific satiety" is the way nutritionists describe the human appetite for different foods. Nature has a way of making sure you eat a varied diet to get the full array of nutrients. That's why trendy food-group-elimination diets rarely work: They literally force you into craving foods your body needs.

In general, Americans' portion-control meters are out of whack.

Watch Your Portions

In addition to adopting a varied, balanced diet—cutting out junk, reining in fat and sweets, and eating more nutritious plant foods such as produce and whole grains—it's important to consume reasonable portions. In general, Americans' portion-control meters are out of whack. Foreigners are astounded at the sheer size of the servings we give ourselves. Imports like the bagel and the croissant have ballooned to double their original size, movie theaters sell mammoth containers of soda and popcorn, fast-food assembly lines crank out "supersize" meals. As our plates grow bigger, so do our girths. And the result is distressing: For the first time in history, the majority of Americans are overweight.

Readjusting portion size doesn't mean pulling out a scale and measuring every serving down to the last gram. It means teaching yourself to stop eating when you're no longer hungry—before you're stuffed. This is particularly important if eating has become an obsession for you. If you consume sensible servings of healthful food and stop when hunger abates, your obsession will ebb, and along with it the guilt that fuels the starve-and-binge cycle. You might find that you're losing weight without following any formal program.

Getting Friendly with Food

If you're going to eat the health-wise way, it's important that you have the right attitude about food, that you never think of it as the "enemy." Unfortunately, that's often the message from diet gurus. Severe diets, people are finally realizing, only make matters worse. The more you deny yourself, the more you wolf down in the end. The solution: Allow yourself to eat and the dieting demons will loosen their hold.

"Food isn't the dieter's problem; it's the solution."

Eat to Satisfy Your Palate

In the words of one weight-loss expert, "Food isn't the dieter's problem; it's the solution." Some dieters have gained control of their waists by abandoning tasteless "lite" foods and the sterile convenience of frozen diet dinners. Eat to satisfy hunger and your palate, these people would advise you; just make sure you stop before you're too full. One thing that might help you push away from the table sooner than in the past is knowing that another delicious meal is right around the corner. You don't have to deprive yourself—especially of flavor—to make a diet work. Indeed, the fresher and more high-quality the ingredients, the easier it is to prepare mouth-watering meals that are low in calories. You can perform magic with a piece of fish when you've got the greenest greens, the reddest peppers, some garlic, and extra virgin olive oil.

That's all well and good, you might say, but what about those secret sinners among us who would sell their souls for a 32-ounce bag of candy-coated chocolates? Cheer up. A lot of chocoholics, potato-chip addicts, and other victims of temporary food insanity have found a clever answer that may help you, too: They keep the pantry stocked with their favorite food, knowing that because it's there, they can decide calmly when and if they really want it—rather than running to the store for a midnight binge. "Scarcity makes people anxious; surplus calms them down," says Jane Hirschmann, coauthor of *Overcoming Overeating*. Some people find that it helps to savor a bite-sized serving of their favorite food every day, knowing that if they denied themselves, they'd be in danger of a frenzied raid on the pantry.

Fill Up without Filling Out

How can we be satiated before we're stuffed? Researchers have discovered that the weight, volume, fiber content, and nutrient makeup of food all help set in motion physiological processes that contribute to the agreeable sensation that follows a sumptuous meal. Foods high in fat are slow to trigger satiation signals because they're low in weight for the number of calories they deliver. You're likely to take in far more calories from high-fat foods than from protein and carbohydrate foods before you feel full. The foods researchers have found to be most efficient at quenching the appetite are fruits, vegetables, legumes, nuts, whole grains, and fish.

High-fiber foods—beans, corn, broccoli, brown rice, apples, dried fruit, and the like—are particularly good at filling you up without filling you out. They pack a lot of volume for their calories, and they hang around in your stomach longer, delaying the time when you feel hungry again. While a three-ounce, 470-calorie cheeseburger fits in the palm of your hand, you'd have to polish off a plate crowded with two ears of corn, a baked potato,

High-fiber foods are particularly good at filling you up without filling you out.

a cup of carrots, and a cup of cooked spinach to approach the same number of calories.

Fruits, vegetables, legumes, nuts, whole grains, and fish. Okay, you might say, but what do you do with these appetite-quenching foods, separate them into bland piles on your plate? Not at all. One of the secrets to getting friendly with food is learning how to use ingredients in mouth-watering combinations. And the combinations from Nature's bounty are endless. The gifts of Neptune? Try your shrimp grilled with garlic and fresh peppers, your scallops broiled with lemon juice and a splash of olive oil. Or try going to a sushi bar. Wondering what to do with those highly touted beans? Puree some chickpeas with garlic, olive oil, and lemon juice and you'll have a creamy hummus spread for rye crackers or celery sticks. Toss some cannelloni beans into a tomato sauce spiced with garlic and minced anchovy, or small bits of prosciutto, then serve it over a smaller portion of pasta than you might otherwise eat. A baked potato without the butter and the sour cream? You obviously haven't sampled the perfection of a spud topped with salsa. A plateful of vegetables? Roast them in a little olive oil and garlic, sprinkled with fresh rosemary or thyme—pure ambrosia by the winter fireplace or on the summer deck. This isn't to undersell the delights of poultry, meat, and other foods. Served as lean cuts and in reasonable portions, lovingly prepared, they can enhance the eating experience without enlarging the waistline. Variety, as they say, is the spice of life.

> Most successful dieters go through a series of stages before reshaping their eating habits.

Do It for Yourself

Variety, moderation, a stocked pantry. Do these avenues to a slimmer waist sound a bit too easily traveled? In truth, people who master the get-friendly-with-food approach often do so after years of trial and error. What starts as a diet slowly morphs into a way of life. Various studies over the past decade have revealed a number of common threads among dieters who have met with long-term success, and one of them is precisely this: No matter how weird or wacky their diet starts out, weight losers eventually adopt a sensible eating plan they're content to stay on for the long haul.

How can you achieve this enviable peace of mind? It isn't easy, according to Daniel Kirschenbaum, a psychologist and director of the Center for Behavioral Medicine in Chicago. Most successful dieters go through a series of stages before reshaping their eating habits. First there's the honeymoon; it's filled with optimism, but that optimism usually fades within a few months to a year. Next comes the frustration stage, when you realize you have to work harder to lose weight and keep it off than people of normal weight. "There's annoyance and anger and a 'Why me?' effect that can last for many months or even years," says Kirschenbaum. Only in the third stage—tentative acceptance—do you come to terms with your lot and achieve a peaceful sense of resolve. "They stop thinking, it's not fair that I have to eat less than my wife who weighs half what I do, or it's not fair that I have to exercise every day," says Kirschenbaum. "They no longer consider their effort a sacrifice. It feels more natural, healthier." Once a person goes from understanding what it takes to actually living it, there's no turning back.

And that understanding comes from within. Have you ever been motivated to lose weight by a snide comment from a spouse or coworker, or by an upcoming event such as a wedding? The problem is that external events can only keep you motivated for a short time. It's when you start shedding pounds for yourself that your weight-loss efforts may finally be rewarded. Like other successful dieters who have turned the corner, you'll stop worrying and learn to love food. Farewell to the self-defeating notion that biology is destiny. Farewell to the binge-and-starve days of yore. No more gorging out of boredom, loneliness, anxiety, guilt, or habit. Food, you'll discover, is one of nature's most marvelous gifts.

When you start shedding pounds for yourself, your weight-loss efforts may finally be rewarded.

Jumpstarting Your Body

If sensible eating is one half of the healthy-living equation, the other half is exercise. Why is it so hard to accept this? In part, it's our busy lives. Some of us can't squeeze an extra minute out of the day to exercise. And in part it's our couch potato culture. People drive to work, take an elevator instead of the stairs, sit at a desk all day, then unwind in front of the tube at night. They may be as mentally agile as astrophysicists, but tell them to exercise and they react as if they're being read a death sentence. For many of us, it just seems like one more chore that we don't have time for.

Make Exercise Part of Your Routine

If you're pressed for time, consider this: Brisk activity will rev up your engine, making you more energetic, more alert, and more productive—perhaps even prompting the discovery that you have more spare time than you thought. The trick is getting launched—once you do, the benefits of exercise will likely get you hooked. Before starting an exercise routine, consult your doctor. Excessive weight is a risk factor for heart disease, as are conditions that often accompany being overweight such as high blood pressure, high blood-fat levels, and diabetes. It's important that you get a stress test to see whether your heart can sustain moderate exercise. It's equally important, if you're a novice, not to overdo it the first day. To avoid overtaxing weak muscles or an ill-prepared heart, ease into exercise. Start with a few minutes each day and build up gradually over several weeks until you've hit your goal. That's the best insurance against heart attack, injury—and the discouragement that can result from an overzealous start.

Once you establish a regular routine, the cascading benefits of exercise may well surprise and delight you—and make you wonder why this epiphany was so long in coming. On top of burning calories, brisk exercise appears to crank up the body's levels of antihunger chemicals: glucose, serotonin, noradrenaline, adrenaline, and dopamine. When you diet, you force yourself to eat less. When you exercise briskly, you want to eat less.

Moreover, physical activity makes you feel better. The hunger-snuffing hormone noradrenaline doubles as a mood-elevating stimulant. After 10 minutes of sustained activity most people, if they're already fit, experience an invigorating high that can last as long as six to 18 hours beyond exercise. And studies have shown that a single 40-minute walk can lessen anxiety. If you find yourself raiding the cookie jar whenever you're blue or tense, regular exercise might be a good antidote.

When you diet, you force yourself to eat less. When you exercise briskly, you want to eat less.

Become a Calorie-Burning Machine

There's yet another compelling reason to exercise. Amino acids replenish the protein that makes up about 30% of your muscle. And exercise enables muscle to absorb amino acids more readily. If you follow a diet without exercise—no matter what kind of diet it is—some of the weight you lose will be muscle. If you return to your old eating habits and still don't exercise, you'll regain weight in the form of fat, not muscle. If you exercise while dieting, however, you'll build muscle and improve your calorie-burning efficiency. Muscle burns many more calories than does any other tissue. Performing the same ordinary activity, a muscle-bound 200-pounder may burn as many as 800 calories more a day than a 200-pound person who is out of shape.

One of the muscles you strengthen while exercising is your heart. It expands like a balloon when filled with blood, then contracts to flush the blood out through your arteries. Sustained activity increases the flow of blood to this organ, raising the resistance it encounters when contracting and making it stronger. The result? Not only greater cardiovascular fitness but also improved capacity for brisk exercise—the only kind that's going to zap pounds and keep them off.

Exercise Longer—or More Intensely

The best exercise for burning calories is aerobic, the sort that makes you feel winded and increases the efficiency with which your heart sends oxygenated blood to your muscles. But weight lifting is also good because it builds calorie-burning muscle. And stretching promotes flexibility and prevents injury. The perennial question is, how much of all of this do you need to do in order to slim down and stay that way? The Surgeon General's "exercise-lite" prescription—30 minutes of moderate exercise most days of the week—has its benefits, not least among them lowering the risk of heart disease and osteoporosis. But researchers are finding that on the road to fitness, exercise lite is your granny's Model T. Those who want a noticeably trimmer body will have to exercise either longer or more intensely. This is not necessarily as daunting as it sounds. You don't have to perform herculean feats to trim your waist. You can do

You don't have to perform herculean feats to trim your waist.

If you exercise while dieting, you'll build muscle and improve your calorie-burning efficiency.

something as easy as walking, as long as you do enough of it. Walking, like swimming, running, bicycling, and any number of other activities that get you winded, is aerobic. Not so very long ago our ancestors lived in nomadic bands of hunter-gatherers, roaming hundreds of miles a month in search of food and shelter. Evolution shaped our legs for walking. Interestingly, of the successful dieters listed with the National Weight Control Registry—a database that tracks people who have lost 30 pounds or more and kept them off for at least a year—49 out of every 50 follow a regular walking routine. The advantages of walking can be irresistible: Not only does it burn calories but it's cheap, convenient, easy on the joints, and almost anyone can do it, either alone or in sociable groups. No definitive study has established exactly how many minutes of walking a day will keep you trim. But ask researchers for their commonsense advice, and over and over you'll hear 45 minutes a day.

For aspiring exercisers who find three-quarters of an hour a long stretch, it helps to know that breaking up the time—say, into three 15-minute walks—burns calories just as effectively as taking one 45-minute walk. And you can get the same results walking five rather than seven days a week, as long as you make up for the no-exercise days with longer walks of an hour a day. Or you can take a vigorous three-hour hike on Saturday and polish off your week's total with 45-minute walks on Monday, Wednesday, and Friday. Exercise, thank goodness, can be sliced and diced any number of ways to fit busy lives.

If you opt for a 45-minute program, how fast will you lose? That depends. A 150-pound person walking 15 minute miles may burn up to 300 calories in 45 minutes. About 3,500 calories equals one pound of body fat. In theory that means this person could lose a pound every 11 to 13 days. Of course, there is no typical 150-pounder, and how fast you lose will depend on your age, starting weight, diet, and metabolism. One person might take months to shed the first five pounds, then lose 20 pounds in six months. Another might lose two pounds a month from the get go.

What if you want to save time and still lose weight? Then exercise harder. "If you make your exercise high intensity," says exercise physiologist Bob Otto of Adelphi University in New York, "you don't have to do it every day of the week, and you can keep it short." According to the American College of Sports Medicine, people working out at a higher intensity—75 to 85% of their maximum heart rate—for 20 minutes may well burn as many calories as a person walking for 45 minutes. Moreover, during the hours following a high-intensity workout, carbohydrates and fat are used up at rates much higher than those following a low-intensity workout.

In addition to aerobic activity like walking, the American College of Sports Medicine recommends resistance or weight training, which builds both bone density—good insurance against osteoporosis—and calorie-frying muscle. People strapped for time can pursue this without too much additional strain on their schedules. Thankfully, the old three-sets-per-lift (or per machine) dogma has been set aside. Every study over the last 30 years has found that doing three sets has no advantage over doing one, as long as you progressively lift heavier weights. Christine Snow and Gianni Maddalozzo, experts in weight lifting in the department of exercise and sport science at Oregon State University in Corvallis, recommend a workout of just six to eight repetitions on five machines—the lateral pull-down, chest press, seated row, leg press, and calf raise. Each machine works three or four muscles, which is why you can use so few. Complete the routine with some abdominal crunches and you've only used up 20 minutes. For maximum benefit, do this on top of your 45 minutes a day of moderate aerobic exercise (or 20 minutes of strenuous aerobic exercise). If you don't have the time, skip the aerobic exercise twice a week and just pump iron on those days. Make sure, however, that you spend 10 minutes warming up your muscles with an activity like walking before hitting the machines or the weights. That will help prevent an injury that could derail your exercise activity for weeks or even longer.

Get Hooked, and Learn the Secret of Lifetime Weight Control

Once exercise becomes a part of your routine, you'll be hooked, and you will have discovered what almost any weight researcher or doctor knows—that exercise is critical not only to your health but also to lifetime weight control. Consider a weight-loss study done at Baylor College of Medicine

What if you want to save time and still lose weight? Then exercise harder.

in Houston. Men and women were divided into three groups: exercise and diet, diet only, and exercise only. Initially, people in the diet-and-exercise group came out ahead. Following a regimen of 1,200 calories daily with exercise three to five times a week, they lost an average of 20 pounds over one year. Those in the diet-only group dropped 15 pounds. The exercisers shed just six. But something strange happened in the study's second year. By the end of that period, members of the exercise-only group had pulled ahead of the pack—not by suddenly dropping untold pounds but by keeping off what they had lost. The two other groups gained back much of the weight they had lost. What was going on?

It may have been that dieting had just proved too difficult to sustain. "It's like asking people to breathe through a straw," says Ken Goodrick, an assistant professor of medicine at Baylor's Behavioral Medicine Research Center and one of the study leaders. "They can do it for a while, but pretty soon they're gasping for air." The frustration and unhappiness of dieting denial can lead to bingeing, and that can end up undermining everything. Which may be why, over the long run, the diet-and-exercise subjects failed to keep up with the exercisers.

Granted, exercise alone is a slow way to lose weight. The calories you burn in a 45-minute walk can be reinstated in a minute with half a piece of apple pie. But the benefits that exercise confers—more energy, less stress, a boost in self-esteem—can ease dieters' low moments, resulting in less bingeing, healthier eating habits and, ultimately, slimmer silhouettes.

Getting hooked on exercise may be the best lifetime weight-loss and maintenance plan around. In the end, it doesn't matter if you're a buns-of-steel 20-something going through your stair-stepping routine at the gym or a grandmother who straps on walking shoes and hits the de facto treadmill at the mall. What matters is getting the body that evolution shaped for motion into motion—and into shape.

What to Look For in Any Diet

The promises put forth by diet crusaders are all too often inflated and, lamentably, much too often convincing. Uncredentialed charlatans aren't the only problem. Even bona fide medical doctors, angling for a big following or the profits from a best-seller, have been known to peddle misinformation and half truths to the unsuspecting public. In the babel of diet books vying for your attention, how can you tell the facts from the fibs and find the diet that's right for you? Just as we did in evaluating the diets included here, a good strategy is to ask the following questions.

What Does It Promise?

It's easy for diet authors to lift sentences from prestigious medical journals, string them together out of context, and make a pet diet program sound like solid science. Some gurus develop a kind of blind faith in these faulty premises. As Dr. Frederick Stare, founder of Harvard University's Department of Nutrition, and Dr. Elizabeth Whelan, president of the American Council on Science and Health, put it in their book *Fad-Free Nutrition*, "What may begin as an innocently flawed idea can swell to an ill-conceived theory, and from there to a full-blown cult." Many fad diet books claim some special knowledge about the nature of food or the way your body processes it. They praise or ban specific foods. Vow that certain foods can change your "body chemistry." Or blame specific hormones for obesity. These should all be warning signs. Plans that promise too much almost always fail to pay off.

Plans that promise too much almost always fail to pay off.

Does the Author Damn the Medical Establishment?

When the questionable theory doesn't jibe with fact, well-established scientific principles are often dismissed. Watch out for messianic diet proponents who vehemently condemn the medical establishment and who, in the absence of clinical trials or reliable statistics to back up their positions, resort to persuasive-sounding case histories and breathless testimonials to win converts. And watch out for those who cite a path-breaking medical study. Was this a preliminary investigation only? How large was the study, and what was its duration? Was it conducted on animals only, or also on humans? Most important, has it been confirmed by follow-up studies? If you find an author citing studies without clarifying such issues, it may be time to shop for another diet.

Trumpet a Revolutionary Approach?

Any book that purports to shatter the inertia of established medical research with a "revolutionary" program or a miraculous "breakthrough" should be approached with caution. Consider the book that launched a well-known low-carbohydrate/high-protein diet back in 1972, *Dr. Atkins' Diet Revolution*. As the Journal of the American Medical Association pointed out, that diet was neither new nor revolutionary, just a variation on a low-carb approach to weight loss that had been around for years. Moreover, the association pointed out, the author's claim that low-carb diets were more effective than conventional diets for weight loss had not been borne out by medical research. Research studies are not conducted overnight, and true scientists do not accept an outcome until it has been proven conclusively. To this day, despite a national epidemic of carbophobia, the superiority of low-carb diets for weight loss has still not been proven. (See also the review of *Dr. Atkins' New Diet Revolution*.)

Guarantee Rapid Weight Loss?

Books that trumpet rapid weight loss are also suspect. While shedding pounds quickly is possible, it is not usually healthy. The typical crash diet results in water loss at first. You'll be a dried bean that plumps back up as soon as you go back to eating as usual. After the first few days or weeks on a low-calorie diet, of course, fat will be lost too, but the only way it can be shed quickly—to the tune of two pounds a week or more—is by starving yourself of nutrients and body fuel. It's healthier to go for slow and steady rather than slam-dunk weight loss.

And the measured approach will improve your chances of success. Realistic diet programs take into account not just the heady

It's healthier to go for slow and steady rather than slam-dunk weight loss.

phase of weight loss but also the post-mortem weight maintenance stage. Weight maintenance is the most difficult part of weight control, and the most sensible diet plans are those that address this phase in earnest, giving advice on permanently altering your eating habits and incorporating exercise into your daily routine.

Vow to Cure All Your Ills?

The more things change, the more they stay the same. In 1898 an ad for Grape Nuts, one of food magnate C. W. Post's products, promised to cure appendicitis, tuberculosis, and malaria, as well as to feed the brain and tighten loose teeth. Some of today's diet crusaders are almost as bold as Post was in advertising their cure-alls. All too often, dietary regimens are presented as possessing the power to ward off disease, snuff out aches and pains, prevent mood swings, and put you on a permanent high. Yes, a diet low in saturated fat may help prevent heart disease. A diet rich in vegetables and fruits may help fight cancer. A diet that moderates carb intake will help tame insulin surges in people with diabetes or the condition known as insulin resistance. A diet that succeeds in motivating you to cast off weight will probably make you feel more energetic. But no single program is a cure for everything—diabetes, hypoglycemia, heart disease, emotional disorders, insomnia, allergies, and so on. Your antennae should go up whenever an author promises or suggests that his or her diet will take care of a laundry list of ills. That person is either deluded or dishonest.

> No single program is a cure for everything.

Is It Healthy?

Being overweight is unhealthy. It raises your risk of osteoarthritis, hypertension, gallbladder disease, diabetes, heart disease, and stroke, and each year causes tens or even hundreds of thousands of premature deaths. But by the same token, dieting to lose weight can be unhealthy. We'll say it again: In addition to a certain minimum number of calories, your body needs a variety of foods and some measure of balance among fat, protein, and carbohydrate. The most recent trend in America is the easy-fix diet that lops off an entire food group. If I cut out carbohydrates—or protein or fat—the reasoning seems to go, I can load up on other foods and still lose weight.

That's unwise. Even if a lopsided diet does help you lose weight at first, stick with it long enough and it may make you sick.

On an extended high-protein low-carb diet you could grow too weak to cross the room. On a long-term low-protein high-carb regimen you could lose your hair or see your fingernails split. And if an unbalanced diet doesn't make you sick, chances are it will make you feel deprived, resulting in bingeing and weight regain. So while you consider the diets reviewed in these pages, do your body a favor. Ask two central questions: Does this program limit calories without sacrificing nutrients available from specific food groups? Is it a healthy guide for lifetime weight maintenance? If the answer to either of these questions is no, you might be better off seeking another program.

Should You Join the Low-Carb Bandwagon?

Despite their critical role in fueling the body, carbohydrates have a bad reputation. In recent years the blame for America's obesity has been pinned primarily on sugar. It's true that Americans are eating more sugar than ever—consumption climbed from 118 pounds per person in 1975 to a whopping 150 pounds in 1995—and that refined sugar is low in nutrients and high in calories, a villain food for would-be weight losers. But if you take a look at the average size of entrees in American restaurants, you'll realize that it's not just sugar that's making us fat. People just eat too much, period, and they don't exercise.

Despite the lack of evidence, many Americans, reassured by gurus expounding eccentric theories, are barreling ahead with radically low-carb diets. These can be dangerous. Aside from zapping your energy and possibly incapacitating you for exercise (remember, carbs are your body's number one fuel), such regimens can deprive you of essential nutrients. Milk and yogurt, for example, pack enough carb to be stricken from the list of allowed foods on a very-low-carb diet, raising the risk of osteoporosis. Fruits and starchy veggies are full of carbs—they, too, are often eliminated from low-carb regimens, raising the risk that you'll be missing out on certain essential vitamins and minerals, including potassium, magnesium, beta-carotene, and vitamins C and E. Carb deprivation can lead to nausea, dehydration, constipation, and loss of muscle tissue. Moreover, ketones, the acidic chemicals formed in the absence of carbs, can upset the acid-alkali balance in the body, raising the risk of coma and death.

The prevailing atmosphere of carbophobia has fostered some misconceptions of which you should be aware. One is that insulin and carbohydrates make you fat. In a normal person, the rise in blood sugar, or glucose, after eating carbs stimulates the pancreas to secrete insulin. Insulin is the hormone that converts glucose into energy for your body's cells. Also, insulin converts excess glucose not needed for energy into fat. In some people, however, the cell receptors for insulin perform less effectively, and the conversion of glucose into energy goes awry. One result of this is that the pancreas secretes more and more insulin.

These people are called insulin resistant. Because insulin-resistant people experience an abnormal insulin surge after eating carbs, and because insulin can indeed turn glucose into fat, some diet crusaders have portrayed carbs as "glucose bombs" and insulin as a "fat-packing hormone." If you eat carbs, they say, you'll get fatter than if you eat an equivalent number of calories in the form of fat or protein. Moreover, they contend, if you're insulin resistant you're more likely to grow fat.

Nonsense, says renowned endocrinologist Gerald Reaven of the Stanford University School of Medicine. "Carbs don't make you fat, and insulin doesn't make you fat. Calories make you fat." Evidence shows not that insulin-resistant people tend to become overweight, but rather that overweight people tend to become insulin resistant. If you lose weight and start exercising, your risk of insulin resistance goes down. A glance at the Chinese will explode the myth that carbs and insulin resistance make you fat. The Chinese consume a high-carb diet of rice, but they're slender (not to mention physically active) and as a rule they don't suffer from insulin resistance.

Another prevailing misconception: Low-carb diets make you lose weight faster or more effectively than other diets. Studies simply haven't borne this out. In one conducted by Reaven, people were put on diets consisting of either 85% or 17% of calories from carbohydrates. "The only thing that affected their weight was how many calories they ate," he says. The percentage of carbohydrate made virtually no difference.

The prevailing atmosphere of carbophobia has fostered misconceptions.

29

What's the Scoop on High-Protein Diets?

The low-carb craze goes hand in hand with high-protein mania. After all, if you cut out carbs you have to make up for the loss of nutrients with either fat or protein, and wouldn't you rather chew on steak than drink oil or swallow butter? In the popular imagination, dietary protein is compact and "lean," while carbs, like the Pillsbury Dough Boy, are squishy and chunky—and your body mirrors what you eat. This cloudy notion is reinforced by quasi-scientific theories put forth by diet crusaders to convince you that you can lose weight faster or more easily on a high-protein diet. There is no evidence to support this. Studies and empirical evidence suggest that when people reduce carbs drastically and graze on as much meat, eggs, cheese, butter, and cream as they want, they do lose weight—but only because their total caloric intake goes down. Apparently, they are not inclined to make up the calorie deficit caused by eliminating carbs—about half the calories in a standard balanced diet—by gorging on protein and fat. High-protein low-carb diets are really low-calorie diets in disguise.

High-protein low-carb diets are really low-calorie diets in disguise.

What dangers lurk in a high-protein diet? If it gives you license to wolf down red meat and other saturated-fat-harboring foods, your LDL could soar, setting the stage for heart disease. Moreover, a diet rich in animal protein could elevate your blood levels of homocysteine, an amino acid that has been linked to heart attacks and stroke as well as Alzheimer's disease. If the diet simultaneously calls for a drastic reduction of carbs, you could experience fatigue, nausea, and dehydration. Other possible complications include hypotension, constipation (meat, poultry and fish aren't fiber foods), and aching legs. Moreover, some experts say that a high consumption of protein is undesirable because the more protein you eat, the more calcium you excrete, which may deplete the bones of calcium. Then there's the liver and kidney connection. Your body can't store protein, so your liver and kidneys have to work overtime to process it, either for elimination or for conversion to glucose or fat. The extra burden on these organs can cause them to enlarge—a dangerous prospect if you have preexisting liver or kidney disease.

These are some considerations you should keep in mind when you browse through the low-carb high-protein diets presented in the following pages. Watch for *Dr. Atkins' New Diet Revolution,*

The Zone, The Carbohydrate Addict's Lifespan Program, Protein Power, The 5-Day Miracle Diet, The Complete Scarsdale Medical Diet, The Schwarzbein Principle, Suzanne Somers' Get Skinny on Fabulous Food and—last but not least—*Sugar Busters!*

Are Low-Fat Diets Smart?

For some people, going low fat is an effective route to weight loss. Whether it works over the long run—preserving your hard-won weight loss—is questionable. In addition to helping you absorb certain vitamins and minerals and performing other vital roles, a moderate amount of dietary fat gives food staying power and keeps hunger at bay. It also makes food palatable. Many people find they can't stick with low-fat diets because they're so boring.

As for the dangers of a low-fat diet, only protein-supplement fasts and true fasts are low enough in fat to pose an immediate risk to your health. Over the long term, however, people who reduce fat intake to 10% of calories or less may end up with a cosmetic deficit: lackluster hair, dull fingernails, or sallow skin. And there's a more serious reason to question the wisdom of making a low-fat diet into a life-long habit. It appears that an extremely low-fat high-carb diet—the sort presented in *Eat More, Weigh Less, The Pritikin Principle,* and *The 20/30 Fat and Fiber Diet Plan*—might actually boost the danger of heart disease. When people go on a low-fat high-carb diet and they don't exercise, says Frank Sacks, an epidemiologist at the Harvard School of Public Health, they tend not to lose weight; their triglycerides go up, and their HDL goes down. They end up worse off than when they began.

Should you get tied up in knots about your fat allowance? No. A sensible target is to get 20 or 30% of your daily caloric intake from fat, depending on your needs and your tastebuds. You might seek out *Choose to Lose* and *Dr. Bob Arnot's Revolutionary Weight Control Program* in the following pages, which offer diets that are moderately low in fat. More important than your total fat percentage, however, is reducing your intake of saturated fat—or replacing it with unsaturated fat. Saturated fat is the skull-and-crossbones clogger of arteries, best limited because it can send your cholesterol soaring. Most experts recommend that you restrict saturated fat intake to 10% of your calories.

If you're going to tally percentages by generally recommended guidelines, that would allow you some 20% of your daily calories from unsaturated fat. And studies indicate that the healthiest unsaturated fat is monounsaturated—the kind found in olive, canola, and peanut oil. That's why you've heard praises sung of the Mediterranean diet, the type of cuisine touted in *Low Fat Lies*. It's rich in olive oil and associated with a low incidence of heart disease.

Does Your Diet Follow the Principles of Balance, Variety and Moderation?

In short, no drastic food-group-reduction diet is healthy over the long run. Plans that are eccentric in other ways—for example, *The Body Code*, which tailors your diet to your so-called body type, and *Fit for Life*, which resurrects century-old notions about food combining—are equally unlikely to promote long-term health. Of course, we can't dictate what sort of program you should follow. You know your body best, and only you can decide how to lose weight. Just remember, it's good to be circumspect in the face of overzealous claims that fly in the face of accepted wisdom. Does the diet depart radically from the recommendations of the Food Guide Pyramid? Beware. And also be cautious of diets that eliminate food groups entirely. Current deprivation diets, whether they are high protein/low carb, high carb/low protein, or low fat/high carb, share a disregard for the principles of sensible lifetime weight control: balance among food groups, variety within food groups, and moderation. Without balance, you could deprive yourself of essential nutrients. Without variety, you could nurture a sense of deprivation that drives you to desperation bingeing and yo-yo dieting.

Are there diet books out there that present a varied, balanced—in short, a sensible—program? Most certainly, although their scientific rationale isn't always solid. In the following pages, you might want to take a look at *Low-Fat Lies, High-Fat Frauds*; *Volumetrics*; *Eating Well for Optimum Health*; *Choose to Lose*; *The Diet Cure*; *Dieting with the Duchess*; and *Weight Watchers' 1·2·3 Success® Plan*.

Losing weight is a matter of taking in fewer calories, burning more, or both. There are many paths to this end. Doesn't it make sense to opt for one of the healthiest?

Diet Reviews

In the following pages you'll find a representative range of America's most popular weight-loss programs, from low carb/high protein to high carb/low fat and just about everything in between. As you sample them, our job is to help you sort the facts from the fibs, the fads from the programs that promote lasting, healthful weight control. Of course, you have a unique body with unique needs. Chances are no single diet regimen will perfectly suit your personality, your medical needs, or your tastebuds. In that case, you might want to cherry pick elements from different programs and devise a master plan all your own.

Much of the information we're giving you about individual diets in *The Promise*, *The Method*, and *The Diet as Lifestyle*, represents the author's own position, without our commentary. *The Promise* serves up the basic principles behind a diet, then lays out any evidence the author has marshaled in support of it. *The Method* tells you how the diet works. Typically, this section includes dietary rules dictating what foods you can and can't eat, and in what combinations; how to time meals and snacks; and the percentage of calories you should get from fat, protein, and carbohydrate. *The Method* reviews physical changes that the author claims you'll notice after adopting the plan. It also mentions any additional steps you're supposed to take, such as keeping a food log, taking vitamin and mineral supplements, or practicing stress-reducing techniques.

In *The Diet as Lifestyle*, you'll discover the author's take on lasting weight-loss control. In almost all of the diets reviewed here, exercise is said to be a key component of weight maintenance. You'll read a lot of overlapping advice about the benefits of stretching as well as aerobic and resistance exercise. On the subject of physical activity the diet authors tend to differ in only one respect: the amount of time you should devote to it each week.

Our job is to help you sort the facts from the fibs, the fads from the programs that promote lasting, healthful weight control.

Once the author's position has been laid out, it's our turn. In *Evaluating the Diet*, we'll alert you to any concerns we have about the basic principles of the plan, its rationale, or the evidence claimed in support of it. In some cases, the rationale is faulty and the diet makes little sense, either from a medical or a nutritional standpoint. In other cases, the rationale isn't entirely scientific but the diet—or part of it—would nonetheless promote good health. And then there are the rare diets that are based on solid, up-to-date evidence, whose conscientious creators care as much about your health as they do about your waistline or their wallets.

Next you'll hear what we have to say about the author's promises. Is the diet a quick fix, or will it nurture you in your effort at lasting weight control (as almost all the authors here vow)? Is it a package of petty regulations that will ultimately defeat you—or a flexible approach that recognizes your unique needs and appetite? We'll lay out the diet's strengths and stumbling blocks as we see them, then tell you whether, to the best of our knowledge, we think this program's for you. If you think it might be and you want further information, see the final section on resources.

Dr. Bob Arnot's Revolutionary Weight Control Program

Dr. Bob Arnot, chief medical correspondent for NBC News and author of *Dr. Bob Arnot's Revolutionary Weight Control Program*, begins with a basic principle: Foods are drugs. By feeding your system the right foods at the right time, Arnot contends, you can utilize their chemical properties to satisfy mind and body while trimming pounds. He criticizes the practice of dieting, which he compares to holding your breath: "You can only do it so long before you have to say uncle." Instead, he proposes, you should fill your stomach with "hard foods," foods that satisfy hunger and keep you feeling full longer, often on fewer calories. Tens of thousands of people have shed pounds and shaped up following the principles of his diet plan, he claims. And he promises it will work for you.

The Promise

Basic principles of the Arnot program

Arnot blasts the low-fat, low-fiber, carbo-loading craze of the 1980s, which he blames for making Americans the fattest people in the industrial world. The logic is based on the fact that nearly all carbohydrates can be broken down into glucose. Arnot maintains that when you stuff yourself with bagels, pasta, and other refined-flour "soft" carbohydrates under the false impression that they are healthy low-fat foods, the glucose level in your bloodstream skyrockets. In response, your body produces more insulin, the hormone that controls the level of glucose in your body. This makes you both sleepy and hungry, particularly for sweets. You eat more carbohydrates to fight the lethargy and satisfy the hunger, which just perpetuates the cycle and expands your waistline.

Arnot wants to rescue you from this quagmire. To keep your glucose levels in check, he recommends the following: Avoid refined carbohydrates that rapidly break down into glucose, steer away from saturated fats, which he says reduce the effectiveness of insulin, and eliminate big meals, which cause insulin levels to spike. Instead, he says, eat smaller meals and snacks composed of "hard foods" at regular intervals. Hard foods, he maintains, take a long time to digest, satisfy your hunger, steady your levels of glucose and insulin, keep your body energized and your mind focused—and make you leaner. Hard foods, according to his definition, include high-fiber foods and whole grains.

The explanation

Arnot argues that if you give your body what it needs when it needs it, you'll eliminate cravings and reduce your caloric intake. Grazing throughout the day on planned and meticulously timed meals—Feedforward Eating, as he calls it—will keep your brain alert during the day and help you sleep better at night while maximizing your control over weight, hunger, and mood. High-fiber foods, particularly soluble fibers that absorb water and expand in your stomach, are the foundation of any successful diet, Arnot says. They make you feel full longer than other foods, have fewer calories, and take more time to eat. His diet consists largely of foods high in soluble fiber such as whole-wheat bread, wheat germ, oat-based breakfast cereals and other low-sugar cereals, dried apricots and figs, brussels sprouts, and beans—lots of beans. Proteins, including soybeans, cottage cheese, milk, chicken, and fish, also play a significant role in Arnot's program because they fill you up and, when coupled with the right carbs, build up stores of the neurotransmitters serotonin and dopamine, which keep you alert and prevent wild mood swings. Satiated, focused, and on an even keel, says Arnot, you'll control your diet instead of it controlling you.

If you give your body what it needs when it needs it, you'll eliminate cravings and reduce your caloric intake.

Evidence claimed

Arnot's book is sprinkled with passing references to scientific studies, but none is central to the theories presented. According to Arnot, the results of eight major studies of the relationship between eating habits and weight in different cultures show that millions of people around the world who eat more actually weigh less. The key lies in what they eat. Arnot maintains that the diets of Crete, Asia and Sonora (a state in northwestern Mexico) are the best, being associated with long life expectancy and a low rate of chronic disease. Like Arnot's plan, each of these diets is low in fat and glucose and high in fiber.

Arnot offers a personal testimonial to back up his claims about the efficacy of his weight control program. He intentionally beefed up, gaining 18.5 pounds of fat, then lost it. The trick, he says, was first lowering his glucose load. After that his motivation soared. Any time he wanted, he claims, he could lose a half a pound a day without feeling lethargic.

Despite the claims of scientific evidence, Arnot offers no hard statistics for the successes or failures of people who've followed his plan.

The Method

How the Arnot program works

The weight-loss stage of Arnot's program is Feedforward Eating. Arnot divides each day into "zones" and offers meal plans for each. Depending on your plans for the day, you decide how you want to feel during each zone and eat the foods that will give you the energy, the calm, or the focus to perform accordingly. The day starts with the critical "power zone." Breakfast begins with a "shot" of protein to jump-start your brain, followed by a super-hard low-glucose carb such as homemade oatmeal, meant to curb your appetite until lunch. After a midmorning snack of protein and more high-fiber carbs, you enter the "loading zone." To avoid afternoon stupor, Arnot recommends a lunch of protein and vegetables. When sweets summon in midafternoon, you've entered the "craving zone." Arnot suggests a snack of slow-burning carbs and protein. The "relaxation zone" starts in the early evening. You should eat a meal that curbs hunger without upsetting insulin levels, such as a whole-wheat burrito with chicken, brown rice, and black beans. Finally you reach the "fat zone," the time when you can do most damage to your waistline by eating before bedtime. If you bed down with a full belly, warns Arnot, you'll spend the night adding to your fat stores. If you must eat something, have a bowl of cereal or some fruit and cottage cheese, he advises—just enough to maintain good blood sugar while sleeping. (For foods high in protein or carbohydrates that meet the requirements of Arnot's targeted plan, see the *Food Content Guide*.)

Arnot simply pledges that if you follow his advice, you'll achieve a "comfortable, livable weight that is in perfect balance with your body's metabolism."

An additional zone, called the workout zone, can be inserted anywhere in your schedule. Certain foods will prep you for exercise. Arnot recommends oats 45 minutes before a workout to increase endurance, or a protein-enriched carbohydrate drink a few minutes before starting.

Once your weight is under control, you adopt the "hard cuisine" of another culture for lifetime maintenance. Arnot doesn't specify stages of weight loss. Nor does he recommend target weights, on the grounds that setting potentially impossible goals for people only leads to misery. Instead, he simply pledges that if you follow his advice, you'll achieve a "comfortable, livable weight that is in perfect balance with your body's metabolism."

What you'll notice

The positive effects of his program, Arnot suggests, are immediate. What you'll notice depends on what foods you eat and when you eat them. In general, he claims, you'll have more balanced moods, no cravings, an alert yet relaxed mind, and while exercising, better endurance.

Additional steps to take

Arnot recommends that you have blood work done to test for high insulin levels. A low-glucose diet should go a long way to moderating insulin, but very high levels can be treated with drugs if necessary. Because the diet could increase your intake of protein by 20% to 25%, Arnot advises that you be tested for blood urea nitrogen to make sure you aren't overloading on protein. He also recommends having your cholesterol and triglyceride levels tested before adopting this diet. Plenty of good sleep increases the levels of serotonin in your brain. If you want to raise them further, he claims, light therapy, negative ion generators, or a drug such as Prozac could help. As always, before starting any diet you should review its risks and benefits with your doctor.

The Diet as Lifestyle

Staying the course

While you're losing weight, Arnot's program allows you to sample a variety of foods that cross international boundaries. But once you've reached your weight goal,

> "Even with a major setback, recovery was easy because I didn't crave foods."

you're to follow the diet of a single culture. His reasoning? No research has been done to prove conclusively that certain foods eaten over a lifetime will prevent specific diseases or promote longevity. Such research has been done, however, on the complete diets of different cultures. Since foods probably interact with each other in ways scientists have not yet discovered, it would seem to make logical sense, according to Arnot, to adopt a particular culture's entire meal package in order to reap its health benefits.

Arnot admits that he's strayed from his program occasionally, especially around holidays or while traveling. When a few extra pounds need to be dropped, he follows his Feedforward Eating plan, taking off extra pounds at will by slotting the right meals into the right zones. "Even with a major setback, recovery was easy because I didn't crave foods and my physiology remained that of fat loss." When you fall off the wagon, follow the basic principles of Feedforward Eating, he advises.

Getting into gear

According to Arnot, even slouches will have so much energy and motivation on this program that they'll gleefully engage in exercise. Arnot recommends "fat-ripping exercises," those that burn lots of calories in a short time or that you can sustain for longer without injuring yourself. His favorite aerobic workouts are biking and hiking, but he also recommends cross-country skiing, stair machines, rowing ergometers, roller blading, treadmills, and long-distance running. Swimming (unless you're fast), aerobic dance, strolling, exercise bikes, and cross-country ski machines are overrated in his opinion, because they pose the risk of injury or don't zap enough calories. Cross-training—different workouts on different days—is a good way of exercising muscles without risking injury or overtraining. You might consider buying a heart monitor to make sure you're exercising in your peak heart rate. In addition to aerobic exercise, Arnot recommends weight training to speed up your metabolism, creating a "fat-burning engine."

Evaluating the Diet

Cautions and concerns

Arnot's theories are neither revolutionary—despite the title—nor based on solid science. There is no evidence for his assertion that "soft" carbs make you fat. Like other trendy carb-bashing books, this one can be misleading. Calories make you fat—whether they come from bagels, beef, butter or beans. And the distinction he strives to make between "hard" (good) and "soft" (bad) foods is confusing. "All hard foods give your intestines a really good workout, burning far more calories than slop and even increasing your metabolic rate," he says. Low-fat yogurt is soft in texture but, according to Arnot, good for you; French bread has a hard crust but, being a refined-flour product, is bad for you, says Arnot. But food chemistry is simply too complex a matter for foods to be conveniently pigeonholed as hard or soft. Furthermore, the notion that hard foods burn more calories than "slop" has little foundation in fact. Your overall health and how much you exercise are far more important than what you eat in determining how many calories you burn during digestion.

Arnot puts much emphasis on the presumed benefits of other cultures' diets, and praises in particular the dietary practices of societies with the leanest, healthiest populations. But his less-than-scientific analysis may not give enough credit to the fact that the people eating these diets tend to lead more active lives than typical Americans; it may be the exercise as much as the diet that's keeping those foreigners fit. One way or the other, the evidence just isn't as definitive as Arnot makes it sound.

Arnot also says you can eat until you're full without worrying about how many calories you're consuming and still lose weight. His answer to the calorie conundrum? Eat bulky foods that make you feel full longer on fewer calories. Or shave off pounds by pumping up the intensity of your workouts. Those approaches might work for you, but remember, calories *do* count. You won't lose weight if you take in more than you burn. Period.

Quick fix or lasting results?

Arnot presents his diet as a lifestyle change, not a crash diet designed to drop pounds in a few days or weeks. Some of his basic principles—reduce fat intake, limit sugar, and eat lots of plant foods and high-fiber foods—are practices generally considered crucial to weight control and a long, healthy life. Whether it's necessary to adopt wholesale the diet of another culture to achieve lifetime weight control is arguable.

Flexible or rigid?

To follow Arnot's Feedforward Eating system you'll have to be obsessive about both food and mood—not to mention the clock: "Feedforward Eating is consuming the right foods in advance of a meeting, a workout, a nap, or concentrated intellectual effort so that you feel and perform exactly as you want." All the close scrutiny, if it doesn't drive your peers and family crazy, might ultimately drive *you* crazy.

To be fair, Arnot isn't tightly prescriptive. He suggests ideas for weight-shedding Feedforward meals, such as oatmeal and cantaloupe for breakfast, without dictating meal plans. And for lifetime maintenance he gives you a choice of cuisine from several different cultures, leaving the choices up to you. This is a general approach, not a detailed roadmap to weight control. In addition to not counting calories, you won't have to haul a scale around with you—the diet, for better or worse, doesn't restrict portions.

Stumbling blocks

Aside from matching your meals to your daily agenda, ditching the Western diet may be the hardest part of Arnot's approach. You'll have to learn a whole new cooking style and adapt your grocery-shopping list accordingly. Arnot admits that in cases such as the Asian diet, ingredients may be difficult to find in the supermarket. And they may be costly.

Is it for you?

Arnot jokes that he should call his weight control program "Dr. Bob's Bike and Bean Diet." Biking and beans were the silver bullet that enabled him to control his own weight. If beans aren't your bag, you might want to substitute another food—or another weight control program. And if you can't live without pizza, bagels, ice cream, candy, and lots of red meat, Arnot isn't for you. People with liver and kidney conditions should avoid this diet owing to its potentially high protein content. For most people without preexisting medical conditions, Arnot's approach with its emphasis on low-fat, high-fiber, and plant foods can be a healthy one. The carb bashing is deceptive: He allows you plenty of nutritious whole-grain products. Cut through the trendy, quasi-scientific talk about hard and soft foods and you'll find a reasonably balanced approach to eating for weight loss.

Resources

Learn all about this dietary program by reading *Dr. Bob Arnot's Revolutionary Weight Control Program* (Little, Brown, and Company, 1997). Additional advice can be found in *Dr. Bob Arnot's Guide to Turning Back the Clock* and *The Breast Cancer Prevention Diet.*

Dr. Atkins' New Diet Revolution

Dr. Robert Atkins, cardiologist by training and author of the runaway bestseller *Dr. Atkins' New Diet Revolution,* is a veteran guru of the low-carbohydrate diet. For 35 years he's been promoting a weight-loss regimen that goes against the grain of the calorie-counting American medical establishment. Under Atkins' plan, dieters severely curb their intake of carbohydrates while digging guilt-free into a high-protein, high-fat cornucopia. Under his personal supervision at the Atkins Center for Complementary Medicine, the author claims, countless thousands of diet-challenged patients have shed pounds permanently without a pang of hunger.

The Promise

Basic principles of the Atkins diet

Carbohydrates—a class of carbon-based compounds that includes sugars, starch, and cellulose—exist in a whole host of foods, from grains, beans, and certain dairy products to some fruits and vegetables. One of the fundamental principles of the Atkins approach is that most overweight people are carbohydrate-sensitive: Their weight problems stem from the *way* their bodies process carbohydrates, he says, not the amount of fat they eat. These individuals, according to Atkins, do not metabolize carbohydrates properly because the hormone insulin isn't doing its job.

When you eat carbohydrates, your blood sugar, or glucose, rises. In response, your pancreas pumps out insulin, which converts glucose into energy for cells. According to Atkins, however, many overweight people suffer from a condition known as insulin resistance, a complex and not-fully-understood disorder that affects how insulin processes glucose. In simple terms, the "resistance" refers to the fact that cell receptors for insulin don't work properly; they "resist" the insulin, thereby interfering with the conversion of glucose into energy. As a result, says Atkins, insulin turns more and more glucose into fat, primarily in the form of triglycerides, which both put on the pounds and may also damage the heart. In what he calls a vicious cycle, the body responds to the inefficient processing of glucose by pumping out more insulin, and if the person continues to eat carbohydrates, even more insulin is produced and the fat continues to build up.

How to slow down the diligent "fat-packing" insulin that's wreaking havoc on your body? Simple, Atkins asserts: Break the vicious cycle by restricting carbohydrates, especially processed junk foods such as frozen pies, cookies, nondiet soft drinks, and ice cream. Indeed, on a low-carb diet, Atkins insists, you can eat even more calories than you were eating before and still begin losing weight. And in addition to shaving off pounds, the author says, his regimen will help your heart by lowering triglycerides.

The explanation

The promise seems paradoxical, that you can eat more and actually lose weight. According to Atkins, the secret is in a biological process called ketosis. If you drastically reduce the amount of carbohydrates you eat to 40 grams or less a day, your body enters ketosis, a state in which it burns fat for fuel. This reduces stored fat in the body and at the same time makes what Atkins calls "an end run around insulin," limiting its production of fat in the first place. For diehard doughnut and pizza addicts, curbing carbs might sound like torture. But supposedly, once your body starts burning fat the craving for carbohydrates abates. And in the absence of carbs, fat-rich foods like cheesy omelets, sizzling steaks and butter-drenched lobster do such a good job of dampening the appetite that—according to Atkins—you will tend to eat *less* fat on his diet than on an austere low-fat regimen.

Evidence claimed

Atkins argues that for millions of years—long before they learned to plant grains and bake bread, much less process colas and candy bars—humans survived on a low-carb diet of meat, fish, berries, fruits, and vegetables. It wasn't until the 20th century that consumption of sugar—the chief carbohydrate culprit—skyrocketed. From 1975 to 1995 alone, per capita consumption of sugar in the United States went from a world-leading 118 pounds a year to over 150 pounds. On the surface, Atkins' insistence that sugar and not fat is the culprit causing obesity appears buttressed by this fact: Between the mid-1980s and the mid-1990s, the percentage of daily calories from fat fell from 40% to 33% in the United States, while obesity rose from 25% to 33%—an addition of 20 million cases. In his clinical practice, Atkins claims, he has personally treated frustrated dieters who were unable to shave off pounds on low-fat, 700-calorie-a-day regimens but found success with this low-carb, higher-calorie diet.

The outside evidence that Atkins marshals begins with a landmark study done in the 1950s, when British researchers are said to have demonstrated that a low-carb diet of 1,000 calories took off weight, whereas a high-carb diet of 1,000 calories gave disappointing results. Another study by the same authors claimed that obese subjects did not shed pounds on a balanced 2,000-calorie diet but did lose weight on a low-carb, high-fat diet of equal calories or more.

The Method

How the Atkins diet works

There are four stages to the Atkins diet: induction, ongoing weight loss, premaintenance, and maintenance. Induction is a 14-day crash course during which dieters may lose anywhere from two to 16 pounds. You enter ketosis by limiting yourself to 20 grams of carbohydrate a day. This stage permits cream and butter, unlimited quantities of eggs and almost all types of meat, fish, poultry, and cheese, but only three cups total of low-carb vegetables such as lettuce, mushrooms, avocados, broccoli, and tomatoes. Skim milk and yogurt are hands off (they pack more carbohydrate than cream does), as are all fruits, breads, grains, and starchy vegetables. In addition to losing weight, you'll be cutting out foods to which you may be either addicted or allergic, such as alcohol, caffeine, chocolate, sugar, and grain gluten.

The next stage is ongoing weight loss, which can last from two weeks to two months. During ongoing weight loss you ratchet up your consumption of carbs gradually, by roughly five grams a day, until you discover the maximum level you're able to eat while continuing to lose weight. Five grams a day isn't exactly a feast. It's the equivalent of 15 almonds, six spears of asparagus, or a half cup of tomato juice. When you stop losing weight, you've reached your max and it's time to ease off on the carbs.

By the time you're five to 10 pounds away from your ideal body weight you're in the premaintenance stage, which can last a few weeks or a couple of months. Now weight should be shed more slowly, less than a pound a week. This is the time to learn what exceptions you can make to your diet—during the course of a week, perhaps adding a slice of whole wheat bread or half a cantaloupe—while still seeing your weight go down. Watch out, says Atkins. You'll be burning less fat, and the appetite-suppressing benefit of ketosis will begin to vanish.

Once you reach your ideal weight (see the height and weight chart in the appendix), you go on a lifetime maintenance diet. Atkins suggests a cautious introduction of larger helpings of healthy carbohydrates, which can include starchier veggies, even an occasional potato, and whole grains such as oats. But you must still restrict sweets to those containing sugar substitutes, and no more than one serving of fruit a day. Now the trick is to find the highest number of grams of carbohydrate you can eat without gaining weight *back*. This probably means navigating somewhere between 40 and 60 grams a day, depending on your metabolism.

What you'll notice

Within two days of induction, Atkins assures readers, your food cravings will abate. Withdrawal from food addictions may cause fatigue, palpitations, headaches, or cold sweats—symptoms that should subside three days into induction. By the third or fourth day you may notice a surge of energy as your blood sugar levels stabilize. Constipation is common the first week, a problem Atkins recommends correcting with bulking agents and vita-nutrients. If you have a medical checkup and blood tests before the diet and after, Atkins maintains, you'll notice a whole slew of health benefits, including stabilization of glucose and insulin levels, plummeting triglycerides, and a drop in your total cholesterol level.

Additional steps to take

To measure the regimen's touted effectiveness and health benefits, you should get blood tests for cholesterol, triglycerides, glucose, insulin, and uric acid both before and after induction. In addition, you're advised to stop taking unnecessary medications, many of which inhibit weight loss. During induction you might want to use test strips that measure the presence of ketone bodies in your urine; these carbon compounds tell you whether you're in ketosis. As you slowly begin reintroducing carbs, the strips are a convenient way of indicating whether you've cranked up your intake too much and stopped ketosis. Last but not least, you're steered toward a virtual pharmacopoeia of nutritional supplements to promote cardiovascular health, boost the immune system, control hypoglycemia (low blood sugar)—and compensate for the acknowledged nutritional deficiencies of this diet.

The Diet as Lifestyle

Staying the course

Atkins' maintenance regimen is a lifetime vow to yourself to hold carbs at bay. If you find that you've gained five or more pounds, you should hustle back to the induction diet and progress as before toward your ideal weight. Once back on track, can you binge? Yes, according to Atkins, as long as you stick with protein/fat foods that "don't unleash a metabolic tidal wave in your body." You'll have to be permanently vigilant about fruit and resign yourself to giving up refined sugar. Dieters can fill the gap with a wide variety of mouth-watering foods, including avocado filled with mayonnaise-based crabmeat salad and fried pork rinds (they're zero carb!) with paté. To nip binge mania in the bud, Atkins suggests taking chromium, L-glutamine and B complex vitamins.

Getting into gear

Atkins recommends that you do a reasonable amount of exercise, not only to trim your silhouette but also to make you feel better, strengthen your heart, and reduce your production of "fat-producing" insulin. "If you're over a hundred," he writes, "call me … to discuss the possibility of your not exercising; the rest of you won't get away with this lame excuse." Aerobic exercise, which increases your heart rate and oxygen consumption, is the best kind, says Atkins. He urges those who haven't been exercising at all to begin by walking ten minutes a day, gradually moving up to at least a half hour every day at a brisk pace. Vigorous aerobic activities such as cross-country skiing, running, swimming, and bicycling bring even better results. Anaerobic exercise like weight lifting doesn't significantly increase heart rate, but it strengthens and shapes the body and makes it easier to maintain an ideal weight—something that almost all diet approaches agree on.

> "If you're over a hundred, call me … to discuss the possibility of your not exercising; the rest of you won't get away with this lame excuse." —Robert Atkins

Evaluating the Diet

Cautions and concerns

Though Atkins' approach is compelling to disillusioned veterans of low-fat regimens, dieters should be aware of logical leaps and misleading assumptions in his explanation. Furthermore, any diet plan that has nutritional shortcomings should raise your concerns, and the Atkins' diet has more than its share.

Despite Atkins' claims that carbohydrates are especially to blame for obesity, the simple fact remains that it is *calories* that turn you tubby—not the so-called fat-packing hormone insulin, or carbs, or even insulin resistance. Indeed, evidence suggests that insulin resistance may be a result, not a cause, of excessive weight gain. Endocrinologist Gerald Reaven from the Stanford University School of Medicine, who himself has devised a moderately low-carb diet for people with insulin resistance, says, "The more you eat and the fewer calories you burn up, the heavier you'll get. The law of thermodynamics hasn't been repealed." In addition, restricting carbohydrates—while it will help regulate your insulin and glucose levels if you're insulin-resistant—won't make you burn stored fat any *faster* than restricting other food types. What about the argument that Americans are eating less fat but are fatter than ever before because of their skyrocketing sugar consumption? Yes, intake of sugar has risen—but so has *total caloric* intake. In the 1990s the average American was eating several hundred more calories a day than in the 1970s. As for the claim that ketosis can curb the appetite, no firm proof exists.

The scientific evidence that Atkins draws on suggesting that low-carb diets take off more weight than high-carb diets of equivalent calories is dated. In subsequent studies, while low-carb diets appeared more effective initially, they proved no more beneficial than high-carb diets after 18 days. The temporary advantage of low-carb diets has been attributed to water loss. (Carbohydrates inhibit water loss, and when they are severely curbed it increases the danger of dehydration.) Over the long haul, why do some people lose weight on low-carb diets? Because they are taking in fewer calories. Carbs make up roughly half of the American diet, and when they are eliminated, people aren't inclined to make up the huge deficit with an appreciable increase in protein and fat. At best, low-carb diets are low-cal diets in disguise.

While promoting his program, Atkins glosses over its dangers. Any regimen that gives dieters a green light to consume saturated fat and cholesterol-rich foods should be suspect. Though on the Atkins diet *total* cholesterol might drop because high triglycerides can plummet, unlimited saturated fat intake can drive up LDL cholesterol. Those at worst risk for heart attack are insulin-resistant people who also have high LDL. Another danger is the sort of severe ketosis that this diet induces, which can lead to fatigue, nausea, vomiting and dehydration. Ketones, the acidic chemicals formed during ketosis, can upset the acid-alkaline balance in the body, raising the risk of coma and death and, for pregnant women, endangering the brain of an unborn child.

Atkins downplays additional pitfalls. Eliminating or drastically reducing whole grains, fruits, and many dairy products can cause nutritional deficiencies that might not be corrected by the author's pharmacopoeia of supplements. Possible complications include osteoporosis, constipation, dehydration, hypotension, overtaxed liver and kidneys (they have to work overtime to process all that protein), and halitosis from ketones being eliminated in the breath. Last but not least, a diet rich in animal protein could elevate your blood levels of homocysteine, an amino acid that has been linked to heart attacks and stroke as well as Alzheimer's disease.

Quick fix or lasting results?

If you believe Atkins' claim, tens of thousands of people under his personal supervision—and some 20 million additional dieters—have achieved permanent weight loss. Unlike other regimens, he says, his is perfectly adapted for lifetime use because it "excludes hunger from the dieting experience." Here's the rub: You'll have to be an ardent carnivore for life, limit foods like fruit, whole grains, and pasta whose health benefits most nutrition experts promote—and look the other way when you see someone eating an ice cream sundae. Sugar, farewell.

Flexible or rigid?

As long as you can drastically reduce carbs, you'll find this diet highly flexible. You can throw out your calorie counter, stock up on butter, eggs, and heavy cream, and let yourself loose in the butcher shop. For better or worse, Atkins gives no specific recommendations about the percentage of calories you should get from protein, carbohydrate, and saturated and unsaturated fats. For the hunger-crazed overweight, this diet might look like a dream come true.

Stumbling blocks

You'll be counting carbs instead of calories. For methodical dieters with lots of time on their hands, this won't be a problem. Nor will trooping to the doctor's for blood tests or testing urine for signs of ketosis. But strict adherence to the diet's script could prove impossible for others. Busy people, especially working parents who cook for more than one, might have to simplify matters by just following the diet's general guidelines.

On top of counting carbs, you'll have to determine the uppermost limit you can allow yourself while still shedding pounds. This might prove tricky. You'll likely reach plateaus where you aren't losing, even though you haven't reached your actual limit. Those who survive to the maintenance stage might find it equally perplexing to figure out how many grams of carbohydrate they can eat without gaining weight *back*. Atkins' program is tailored to the individual metabolism—and it's up to the individual to puzzle out the nitty-gritty of ketosis, cholesterol counts, and carb levels.

Is it for you?

If, like so many obese people, you have insulin-related disorders, a low-carb high-protein diet will help you tame the insulin and glucose roller-coaster. And *if* the diet is low enough in calories, it will also help you take off weight. But beware of Atkins' reassurances about the safety of assuaging hunger with foods heavy in saturated fat and cholesterol. Even Atkins admits that roughly one in three people achieves a better cholesterol count on a low-fat than on a high-fat diet. You might consider a low-carb diet that also restricts saturated fats, or better yet, that restricts saturated fat *and* allows a more liberal daily helping of nutritious carbs. (See the diet review of *Protein Power*.) In any event, *don't* follow the Atkins diet without first having a tête-à-tête with your doctor, especially if you're on diuretics or insulin. This regimen is not for people with gout, kidney disease, osteoporosis or type I diabetes, or for pregnant women. And if you're a committed vegetarian, forget it.

Resources

For more on the regimen, pick up a copy of *Dr. Atkins' New Diet Revolution* (Avon Books, 1999) at your bookstore. Atkins' line of vita-nutrients and low-carb food products can be purchased by calling 800-6-ATKINS. To subscribe to his monthly newsletter, *Dr. Atkins' Health Revelations,* call 800-981-7162. If you would like a personal nutritional consultation, either by phone or in person at the Atkins Center for Complementary Medicine in Manhattan, call 888-ATKINS-8. Additional information can be found on the Atkins Center website at www.atkinscenter.com.

The Body Code

Jay Cooper, wellness director of the Green Valley Spa in St. George, Utah, has lived the principles he explains in *The Body Code*. Formerly overweight and an admitted "couch potato," Cooper transformed himself into a marathon runner, triathlete, and fitness trainer through an approach to dieting and exercise he developed over a number of years. Fundamental to his strategy is the notion that no single diet will work for everyone. He classifies people according to body shape, metabolism, and what he calls their energy profile, then tailors a specific nutrition and fitness program for each of four main types. According to Cooper, satisfied clients at the Green Valley Spa have lost weight and turned fit on his customized programs; in *The Body Code*, he offers his lessons to a general audience.

The Promise

Basic principles of the Body Code

Why do some people stay slim no matter what they eat, while others always fight the battle of the bulge? The answer, says Cooper, lies in your genes, which he claims not only determine physical characteristics such as eye color but also your body shape, your personality, and your metabolism—attributes that together make up your body type. You can either work with your body type and achieve lasting weight-loss and fitness results, or grate against it and suffer repeated failure.

> Why do some people stay slim no matter what they eat, while others always fight the battle of the bulge? The answer, says Cooper, lies in your genes.

The key, according to Cooper, is to figure out what body type you are and follow customized guidelines for eating and exercise. He describes four types: the "warrior," who has a substantial upper body, shortish neck, and sturdy, square features; the "nurturer" (women only), with a more prominent lower body, thinner neck, and heart-shaped head; the "communicator," lanky and long, with an oval-shaped head and bony hands and feet;

and the visionary, who has a youthful-looking, less-developed physique and medium-to large-sized head.

Body shape is only one element defining each type; personality traits, favorite foods, and—perhaps most instructive for dieters—where excess body fat tends to show up first also identify each type. According to Cooper, the warrior has an assertive, task-oriented personality, and excess fat collects mostly on the upper body. When "in balance"—that is, feeling fit and healthy, warriors eat starchy vegetables, grains, meats, and lean dairy products; out of balance, they prefer fats, meats, salt, flour products, and alcohol. Nurturers tend to be compassionate and extroverted, and gain weight first in the thighs and buttocks; in balance, their favorite foods are fruits, most vegetables, and spices, while out of balance they tend toward greasy foods. Communicators are creative and verbal with perfectionist tendencies, typcially gaining weight first amidships in the form of a spare tire. In balance, their favorite foods are supposedly proteins, vegetables, and grains; when unbalanced, says Cooper, they make a beeline for sugar, flour products, and caffeine. Finally, visionaries are calm, introverted, and idealistic; gain weight evenly all over the body; prefer cooked vegetables and proteins when in balance, and tend toward sweets, grains, and flour when out of balance.

The explanation

Cooper bases his body typing on several different theories. One of these, first developed in the 1940s and 1950s, proposes that there are three basic anatomical types: mesomorph (average build), endomorph (bulky), and ectomorph (slight). An even earlier theory, dating to the turn of the century, had drawn a connection between body shape, personality, and the endocrine system, which consists of glands throughout the body that release hormones to perform specialized tasks. Cooper combines and elaborates on these hypotheses. Each of us, he says, is born with a dominant gland—adrenal, gonad, thyroid, or pituitary—that determines our body chemistry and metabolism. The adrenal gland controls appetite and reactions to stress; the gonads oversee growth, sexuality, and reproduction; the thyroid directs metabolic rate and energy use; and the pituitary or "master gland" governs all the other glands. And, according to Cooper, each type of gland gets nourishment and stimulation from particular foods. One gland, for example, might respond more to protein, another to carbohydrates, and another to fats.

Here's where things can go wrong, says Cooper. Your dominant gland causes you to crave foods that stimulate it but that will also throw your body chemistry out of whack if you're not careful. These foods are, in his scheme, the very ones you should avoid. Instead of pandering to your dominant gland, Cooper advises, eat foods that stimulate the other three glands and thereby balance your endocrine system.

A further element of Cooper's system draws on the ancient Indian practice of Ayurveda, in which people are classified by underlying energy patterns, or doshas. The three doshas are vata, which regulates movement, pitta, which controls metabolism, and kapha, which oversees structure. By eating certain herbs and foods and practicing specific movements, you can bring the doshas into balance. Knowing your dominant dosha—which, in Cooper's theory, is linked directly to your body shape and your dominant gland—will guide you in the use of meditation and massage for good health.

Evidence claimed

Cooper's evidence is based on personal observation rather than clinical trials or established science. Before going to the Green Valley Spa, he worked with thousands of clients in a wellness program he helped found, taking weekly body measurements and skin-fold calibrations. He would start clients on the same diet and exercise program, then find that their results varied widely. Some lost four to seven pounds a week on a low-fat, high-carbohydrate regimen, while others actually gained weight and felt poorly. The experience helped him confirm and quantify the fact that people are built differently, store body fat in different areas, and lose weight at different rates. Cooper began categorizing his clients by dominant endocrine glands and adjusted their diets accordingly. His new approach, claims Cooper, enabled people to lose weight more predictably than before.

The Method

How the Body Code works

The first step is to fill out Cooper's questionnaire and determine your body type. For each type Cooper designates "plenty" foods, those that can be eaten freely (though within reason), "moderation" or occasional foods, and "seldom" foods. When you're just starting out or if you have a lot of weight to lose, it's best to stay away from seldom and moderation foods and concentrate on plenty foods. To help you plan menus, Cooper includes in his book a selection of recipes developed at the Green Valley Spa. (See "Basic principles of the Body Code", above, for specific foods to eat and to avoid for each body type.)

Cooper's eating plan can be quite specific, as is readily apparent in his prescription for communicators. The communicator will lose weight and stay healthy, he says, by eating lots of leafy vegetables, monounsaturated fats, and lean protein, including all white meats, nonfat dairy products, eggs, some nuts, and soy protein. Green Valley Spa recipes geared toward communicators include such dishes as Spanish egg frittata, spinach fruit salad, and turkey burgers. The communicator is encouraged to eat several small meals throughout the day and to stick with protein for snacks, which, Cooper maintains, will prevent energy fluctuations and mood swings. Communicators are more likely to lose weight if they avoid carbohydrates before noon, eat protein every four hours, and avoid flour, sugar, and caffeine.

What you'll notice

Cooper doesn't say how much weight you can expect to lose, nor does he get specific about how long it will take. But he does claim that his food plans "will bring your body chemistry back into balance quickly enough to give you a noticeable benefit in how you feel and how you look." As an example, he points to one client, who had been plagued by mid-afternoon blood sugar "crashes" all her life. She found she had been eating too much carbohydrate too early in the day and not enough protein. Now, after a year and a half of following Cooper's eating plan, she has more energy than ever before—and no more crashes.

When you start following the Body Code's exercise regimen (see "Getting into gear," below), you may notice a dramatic new sense of well-being—a result, says Cooper, of the release of brain chemicals called endorphins and enkephalins.

Additional steps to take

Cooper suggests that you soak up several hours of sunlight every week, get lymphatic massages, take vitamin, mineral, and herbal supplements, meditate, and practice yoga breathing. Besides increasing oxygen flow through your body, he claims, yoga breathing can calm you down so that you're less likely to overeat out of anxiety. To suppress appetite Cooper also recommends fiber-rich alfalfa or kelp as well as flaxseeds sprinkled over your food in the evening. Cooper says that, unlike other diets, body coding doesn't require a battery of medical tests at the outset.

The Diet as Lifestyle

Staying the course

Cooper is chock-full of advice about remaining focused on his diet. When you lust for "seldom" food, drink cool water and head out for a walk. If you're a communicator, you should avoid large meals, caffeine, and carbohydrates in the morning to control your cravings. More than one of the body types have to give up refined white pasta; if you're one of them, Cooper suggests that you make the switch gradually, adding a little more whole wheat pasta to the pot every time you cook until you're accustomed to the taste. Flaxseed, fennel seed, herbal tea, and sesame oil (you massage your gums with it) are all said to help you regulate your appetite.

Getting into gear

When it comes to exercise, Cooper is very clear on one point: You can't just follow his eating guidelines and expect to lose weight. You need to work your body too. You also have to do specific workouts for your type, which means getting addicted to exercise. Cooper eases you into it with 10 to 20 minutes of walking once or twice a week, ushering you through six stepped levels of aerobic activity until you're exercising between 30 and 60 minutes three to six times a week. To get the maximum benefit from aerobic exercise, Cooper stresses, you have to "find the flow," the point at which you reach "the euphoric high that enables you to run...or cycle...or swim for literally hours."

> When it comes to exercise, Cooper is very clear on one point: You can't just follow his eating guidelines and expect to lose weight. You need to work your body too.

What warriors need most is cardiovascular conditioning, says Cooper. He maintains that warriors sweat a lot and get red in the face when they work out; for them, water sports are particularly helpful. For nurturers, the key to reining in pounds is aerobic activity in a social setting—among other things jazz dance, swim exercises, in-line skating and cycling with a partner. Communicators need moderate but frequent aerobic activity, Cooper says. To prevent boredom they should cross-train, alternating, for example, among in-line skating, Tai bo, mountain biking, rowing, and running. Visionaries require less physical activity than other types but need to exercise regularly to stay balanced and avoid sluggishness. According to the author, the best activities for visionaries are weight-bearing exercises such as walking, jogging, in-line skating, and stair-stepping. All four types should add short bursts of activity to the basic workout once or twice a week.

Evaluating the Diet

Cautions and concerns

Some of the advice in *The Body Code*—about eating and about exercise—is fundamentally healthful. And the recipes Cooper includes emphasize fresh, unprocessed foods that tend to be low-fat. That's the good news. Unfortunately, though, Cooper's entire body-typing approach rests on a flimsy foundation. There just is no valid scientific evidence suggesting that individuals have "dominant" endocrine glands, that body shape is irrevocably determined, that people's personality traits and eating habits are directly related to body type, or that there is an ideal diet for each of the body types described in this book.

Cooper leaves just enough "wiggle" room in his typing to make it seem to work: Visionaries, for example, can be either reserved and introverted or witty and extroverted. So if you have the visionary's body shape, you're almost sure to find in yourself a confirming personality trait. The same holds true for how he relates eating habits to body type. For instance, warriors can crave either lean foods or fatty ones; the difference depends on whether they're in or out of "balance"—a state of being that in essence defines itself.

Thus, Cooper's dietary rules—especially the more unusual ones such as no carbs before noon for communicators, no popcorn for visionaries, no salt for warriors, and virtually no red meat for nurturers—have no reliable evidence supporting them. For each of the four body types the main dietary challenge, says Cooper, is avoiding foods they crave. This approach ignores what nutritionists call "food-specific satiety," that is, the human appetite for different foods. Not all cravings are bad: Often they signal that your body needs something such as the iron in red meat or the energy-packing carb in a plate of pasta. Cravings can be nature's way of making sure you eat a varied diet to get the full array of nutrients.

Depending on your dominant gland, Cooper holds, you might need more protein, or fat, or carbohydrate. This is perhaps the riskiest element of Cooper's scheme—an approach that could lead you to eat unhealthfully. If you have no medical conditions requiring a special diet, the healthier—and happier—road to weight loss is to eat a diet that embraces all three food groups, fat, carbs, and protein, in balanced proportion while reducing your caloric intake and engaging in regular exercise. In fairness to Cooper, he does make a strong case for exercise, the cornerstone of any weight-loss and maintenance regimen. And some of his "seldom" foods are ones that most people are better off consuming in moderate amounts anyway, such as sugar, refined-flour products, junk food, and alcohol. But the whole package just doesn't add up.

Quick fix or lasting results?

Cooper's eating and exercise plan is a "lifestyle modification program" that, he says, is not going to happen overnight. Stick with it and you'll lose weight. So he does promise lasting results. But Cooper wants you to adjust your intake of fat, protein, and/or carbohydrate based on an unsupported theory. Take his path for a lifetime and you may end up with a nutritional deficit from an unbalanced diet.

Flexible or rigid?

Despite Cooper's insistence that you keep strictly to the diet for your type, there's no calorie counting in his approach, and you don't have to haul out the scale to fix portions, so the plan does have flexible features. If you happen to like the "plenty" foods for your genetic type, you can go to town. And "seldom" foods, as the label suggests, aren't completely banned except when you're starting out.

Stumbling blocks

It may be difficult to incorporate Cooper's exercise requirements into your schedule. Cooper admits that "five to ten hours a week can be discouraging" to sedentary types. Also, the fine-tuned vitamin and mineral regimen could be daunting. Supplements are either eaten with lunch, delayed until two hours after lunch, or taken both morning and evening.

Is it for you?

If you have gobs of time for exercise and you don't mind drastically limiting the foods you long for, Cooper's diet might work for you. But you'll have to sign on to his theory that eating your favorites throws your system out of balance and increases cravings. And beware if the plan for your supposed type would lead you to unhealthful eating (see "A Guide to Good Dieting" at the beginning of this book for more advice). Nonetheless, faithfully working out and following the recipes included in *The Body Code* are a surefire way to lose weight: The exercise is intense and the recipes are mostly low calorie. The question must be whether you really need to follow the intricacies of the Cooper approach. The simple truth remains that the fewer calories you pack in your mouth and the more you burn off, the more weight you shed.

Resources

The Body Code: A Personalized Wellness and Weight Loss Plan Developed at the World Famous Green Valley Spa, by Jay Cooper, M.S., with Kathryn Lance, is published by Pocket Books (1999). In the appendix Cooper supplies phone numbers for purchasing exercise equipment, videos, motivational tapes, organic food sources, and alternative health care products. Log on to www.JayCooper.com to find out more about metabolic body types.

The Carbohydrate Addict's Lifespan Program

Although the husband-and-wife team of Richard and Rachael Heller did not invent the term carbohydrate addiction, they are the crusaders most closely associated with it, thanks to a string of best-selling books on the subject. The latest in that line is *The Carbohydrate Addict's Lifespan Program: A Personalized Plan for Becoming Slim, Fit, and Healthy in Your 40s, 50s, 60s, and Beyond*. According to the authors, most weight problems result from people getting "strung out" on carbohydrates. The authors came to this conclusion through their own research and experience. Both Hellers hold PhDs and other advanced degrees. Rachael is a psychologist, Richard a research scientist. Although now retired, they once taught and conducted nutritional studies at New York's Mount Sinai School of Medicine and the Department of Biomedical Sciences at the City University of New York. Their "lifespan program," the Hellers promise, will help you conquer your carbohydrate addiction and cast off unwanted pounds.

The Promise

Basic principles of the Lifespan Program

The Hellers' approach is based on the premise that up to 75% of overweight people (and as many as 40% of those whose weight is normal) are addicted to carbohydrates. According to the Hellers, carbohydrate addiction is a matter not of willpower, but of biology: "You are no more to blame for your condition than you are for the color of your eyes, or your skin, or your hair." Fortunately, they say, you can overcome the addiction, but first you have to take care of the cause: excessive insulin levels. Their "lifespan program," the Hellers promise, will help you normalize your wayward insulin, enabling you to control your carb cravings and hence your weight. If you become a faithful follower, moreover, you'll reap a bonus, they say, reducing your risk of many killer diseases, including heart disease, diabetes, and some forms of cancer.

The explanation

The Hellers' theory starts with some basics about how food fuels the body. When you eat carbohydrate-rich food—such as breads, pasta, sugar, and starchy vegetables—your blood sugar, or glucose, rises. The hormone insulin is responsible for converting that glucose into energy for your cells to use. Any extra glucose is turned into blood fat (triglycerides), which is carried to your fat cells and stored for future use. One important factor in the Hellers' analysis is the claim that insulin actually encourages you to eat carbohydrates by making them taste good; it's the body's way, they say, of getting you to eat the kind of food that can readily be converted into energy.

According to the Hellers, carbohydrate addiction occurs when your bloodstream is flooded with too much insulin. As they put it, the normal workings of insulin go "overboard," and the process of glucose storage goes awry. This produces a cascade of negative effects. First of all, say the Hellers, because insulin makes carbs taste good, you crave them even more when insulin levels are high, and if you take more carbs in, your body must produce more insulin to handle the load. Secondly, when the body detects too much insulin, cells actually "shut down" to it. This is known as insulin resistance, a term that refers to the fact that cell receptors for insulin resist the hormone, preventing it from doing its main job of converting glucose into energy. (For more information on insulin resistance, see the review of the Atkins diet). The authors write, "Since insulin cannot get enough of the blood sugar into organs and muscles that need it, insulin acts as if the blood sugar remaining in the bloodstream is excess." As a result, too much glucose is taken out of the bloodstream and converted directly into fat.

One surefire sign of carbohydrate addiction, say the Hellers, is if you suffer the symptoms of hypoglycemia, or low blood sugar, a couple of hours after eating. These symptoms include feeling unenergetic, shaky, confused, and irritable: Your body is not getting the energy it needs to function properly because glucose levels have plunged in response to malfunctioning insulin. Also, although your body is actually gaining weight as glucose is converted into fat, the authors claim, it thinks it is starving and so drives you to eat more food, especially high-carb snack foods and sweets. Compounding the problem, according to the Hellers, is the fact that insulin resistance increases with age, which is why maintaining an ideal weight becomes harder and harder with each passing year.

Evidence claimed

Numerous scientific studies, say the Hellers, support their observation that "millions of people in this country have a physical imbalance that makes their bodies respond abnormally to carbohydrate-rich foods." They list studies in their bibliography and also cite their own research. To counter skeptics who doubt that people can be addicted to carbohydrates, the Hellers point to research they did that supposedly shows how carbohydrate craving meets criteria for addiction set down by the American Psychiatric Association. Among these criteria are increased use of a substance over time and continued use of a substance despite a desire to stop.

As evidence that their program works, the Hellers point to their own personal experience. Both say they struggled for years with carbohydrate craving and weight problems. Finally, through trial and error, they conquered their addiction and shed excess weight for good (165 pounds in Rachael's case). Later, the Hellers took their hard-won dietary guidelines to Hollywood to help unnamed stars who, it is said, were also enslaved to carbs. The Hellers claim that most of these celebrities found "freedom and success" with their program.

The Method

How the Lifespan Program works

The program consists of two parts: the basic plan, followed by a phase where you choose "options for life." Both are aimed at helping you reduce insulin levels and thus carb cravings. The Hellers recommend that you go on the basic plan for two weeks, then begin adding options one at a time.

The basic plan has three guidelines. First, you eat a balanced "reward meal" every day. This meal should include equal amounts of nonstarchy vegetables (such as leafy greens, green beans, and cauliflower), protein (meat, fish, cheese, eggs, or tofu), and carbs (from breads and pastas to snack foods and sweet desserts). You can have seconds—as long as you eat seconds of everything and in the same equal portions. You must, however, complete your reward meal within one hour (guideline #2). And at all other meals you're allowed only protein and veggies, no carbs (guideline #3). These are referred to as "craving-reducing meals." To help launch you on carb-free cooking, the Hellers offer sample recipes and two seven-day menu plans (one for vegetarians).

Once a day you can eat any of the carb-rich junk food you love, and in any amount. The Hellers claim that by limiting the frequency rather than the amount of such foods you eat each day, you'll lower your insulin levels, subdue your cravings, and lose weight.

The Hellers claim that by limiting the frequency rather than the amount of such foods you eat each day, you'll lower your insulin levels, subdue your cravings, and lose weight.

Two weeks into the program, you begin adding options as you like while continuing the basic plan. The nine options include taking chromium supplements (said to help balance insulin levels), increasing your activity level, reducing sugar substitutes (which, they say, boost insulin levels because they lead your body to expect an influx of sweets), and timing when you use over-the-counter medications. The Hellers claim that each of these options will help tame your insulin levels.

What you'll notice

Within a few days of starting the basic plan, the Hellers assure you, your longing for carbs will have vanished. If you're still salivating at the thought of a doughnut or baked potato, then you may be eating carbohydrate "act-alikes" at your craving-reducing meals—foods and beverages such as sugar substitutes and wine, which can increase cravings and hunger just like carbs themselves. Double-check your menu, the Hellers counsel.

Supposedly, once your cravings are gone, your moods will be less volatile. No more headaches, irritability, fatigue, or other symptoms of low blood sugar, promise the Hellers. If you have hypoglycemia it will disappear, they claim, because your blood sugar levels will no longer be plummeting two hours after eating.

According to the authors, you should also be losing weight at a "satisfactory" rate—between one half and two pounds a week. If not, you may be sensitive to "borderline carbohydrates" such as sausage (a food often classified as meat but containing carbohydrates in the form of grain). You'll need to ban these foods or limit them to your daily reward meal.

Over the long term, the Hellers maintain, you should see a reduction in some of the risk factors for heart disease such as high blood pressure and high triglycerides. You'll also be less likely, they claim, to develop diabetes, gout, and certain types of cancer.

Additional steps to take

To determine the strength of your addiction, the Hellers recommend that you take their 15-question quiz. The only alternative, they say, is to have your doctor administer a five-hour glucose-tolerance test—an expensive, exhaustive procedure, and unreliable unless it is performed more than once, the Hellers say.

The authors also recommend that you weigh yourself at the same time and under the same conditions each day. Keep track of the results and at the end of seven days, they advise, figure your average weight for the week. Use that weight to determine whether you should add more options—which, they say, should further tame your insulin and keep the pounds molting.

The Diet as Lifestyle

Staying the course

To keep on track, the Hellers recommend, you should choose a realistic weight goal, one based on your age, body build, and lifestyle. You should also be aware of any foods or substances that trigger cravings, such as sugar substitutes or monosodium glutamate (MSG); these triggers might make your weight suddenly jump up several pounds. If this happens, don't panic, they counsel; just avoid the trigger and those extra pounds will quickly vanish. Should your weight begin a slow, stubborn climb, simply add an option or two to the basic plan.

Getting into gear

Though exercise is one of the lifespan program's nine options, you don't have to take up running or power walking unless it suits you. According to the Hellers, burning calories is not as vital to weight loss as lowering insulin levels, and moderate or even mild exercise is all that's needed to help keep those levels down. As little as 15 minutes of easy walking three times a week is enough, they say.

Reducing stress is another lifespan option. Stress hormones raise insulin levels, say the Hellers, which drive carb addicts to raid the pantry. Techniques to remove or reduce stress include jogging, getting together with friends, yoga, and warm baths.

Evaluating the Diet

Cautions and concerns

Like other carbophobic diets (see reviews of the Atkins diet, *Protein Power*, and *SugarBusters!*), this one is based on a kernel of truth blown out of proportion. To begin with, while it's true that some people may crave carbohydrates, there is no confirmed evidence that people can actually become physically addicted to them as the Hellers claim. Although they cite studies, their own research has not passed the muster of peer review. Nor is there reliable evidence that insulin abnormalities make people fat. It tends to be the other way around: Overweight people develop insulin abnormalities such as insulin resistance; that is, their insulin levels soar in response to carbohydrate consumption. This calls for a reality check: Weight loss and exercise are more important than the dietary percentage of carbohydrate in treating insulin resistance. Weight loss allows cells to "recognize" insulin more easily, so that less is required. And regular exercise causes insulin to bind more readily to muscle cell receptors, which improves glucose uptake. In other words, weight loss and exercise both enhance insulin sensitivity, and enhanced sensitivity leads to lower insulin levels.

The Hellers seem to imply that more than half of the U.S. population is insulin resistant. Wrong. Studies show that the condition afflicts only 10 to 25% of the population. They also assert that there are millions of carb addicts suffering from hypoglycemia, or dangerously low blood sugar. On the contrary, the American Diabetes Association and the Endocrine Society have issued a joint statement indicating that hypoglycemia has been greatly overdiagnosed. It is now considered a rare condition, usually a complication of diabetes.

Without a solid scientific rationale for this program, dieters might want to think twice before following it. Anyone who truly does have insulin resistance would benefit from an exercise regimen more rigorous than the Hellers' go-light recommendations. In addition to improving insulin sensitivity, exercise—despite the authors' claim—can make or break a weight-loss program. It also lowers the risk of heart disease, and that's an important consideration for anyone consuming the Heller version of a high-protein diet. This plan permits you to graze with abandon on high-fat meats, dairy products, and saturated oils. Because high-fat diets have been linked to heart disease as well as obesity and certain cancers, most experts recommend that you restrict fat to 30% of your calorie intake, with heart-risky saturated fat making up only 10%. On the lifespan program, it would be easy to exceed these limits.

While it is a good idea to reduce carb-loaded junk food in your diet and eat plenty of fresh vegetables, as the Hellers recommend, they offer no compelling reason for drastically reducing carbohydrates in general, limiting them to a single meal, or eating them in equal ratio to protein and veggies at that meal.

A final warning: Low-carb high-protein diets can cause dehydration, constipation, hypotension (low blood pressure), and fatigue. They are also thought to promote osteoporosis and exacerbate liver and kidney disease.

Quick fix or lasting results?

Although the Hellers promise that you'll conquer your cravings quickly, don't expect to be shopping for smaller sizes anytime soon. Given its devil-may-care attitude toward high-fat foods, the lifespan program won't have you shedding pounds rapidly unless you also substantially reduce the calories you consume. If you do shed pounds, will you keep them off? Perhaps—but there are healthier, more sensible lifetime diets that could give you the same results.

Flexible or rigid?

No calorie counting or worrying about portion control, except during reward meals. The rigid aspect of this program lies in its most-unsupported regulations. Each reward fest must consist of equal parts protein, nonstarchy vegetables, and carbs, while other meals have to be carb-free. And the Hellers warn against impulsively switching the time of your reward meal. For example, you're not supposed to eat carb-rich pancakes for breakfast unless you've scheduled breakfast as a reward meal. They offer the least in the way of evidence for how such an approach actually works.

Stumbling blocks

Since they are in a multitude of the foods you eat—not just bread, pasta, and rice but also fruit, dairy products, and starchy vegetables—eliminating carbs from all but one of your daily meals will take considerable self-control and planning. You'll have to learn the art of preparing carb-free cuisine, develop the appetite for it, and if you're cooking for others, convince them to share your deprivation.

There are no limits to how much food you eat on this diet—or how much fat. Thus you'll have to be vigilant about not overeating, particularly at your daily reward meal. After all, calories do count, despite the Hellers' claims.

Is it for you?

If you're insulin resistant or have diabetes, speak to your doctor before going on this diet. The same holds true for people with heart disease or risks for it, since this regimen is potentially high in heart-damaging saturated fat. Pregnant women and people with osteoporosis, kidney or liver disease, or gout should avoid this high-protein diet. It is only for those firmly committed to the notion that reducing carbs and eating high-fat protein will kill cravings and slough off fat. If you're one such hearty soul, check with the doctor first—and remember, watch those calories.

Resources

For more information about the Hellers' program, pick up a copy of *The Carbohydrate Addict's Lifespan Program: A Personalized Plan for Becoming Slim, Fit, and Healthy in Your 40s, 50s, 60s, and Beyond* (Plume, 1998), *The Carbohydrate Addict's Healthy for Life* (Plume, 1996) or *The Carbohydrate Addict's Diet: The Lifelong Solution to Yo-Yo Dieting* (New American Library, 1993). The authors have also written several companion volumes, including *The Carbohydrate Addict's Cookbook: 250 All-New Low-Carb Recipes That Will Cut the Cravings and Keep You Slim for Life* (John Wiley, 2000). People worried about heart disease might want to try *The Carbohydrate Addict's Healthy Heart Program: Break Your Carbo-Insulin Connection to Heart Disease* (Ballantine, 1999). You can find more information about the lifespan program—and participate in an online support group and chat room—through the Hellers' official website at www.carbohydrateaddicts.com.

Choose to Lose

Dr. Ron Goor, a diet and heart disease expert, and his wife, Nancy Goor, a writer and recipe designer, blame America's expanding waistline on dietary fat. Dr. Goor earned his PhD at Harvard and his masters in public health at the Harvard School of Public Health. He coordinated a landmark study undertaken by the National Heart, Lung and Blood Institute (part of the National Institutes of Health) demonstrating that a reduction in blood cholesterol levels decreases the risk of heart attack. He also directed a national program dedicated to educating the public about the health risks of a high-fat diet. Ron Goor's professional involvement in the study of cholesterol and Nancy Goor's development of hundreds of low-fat recipes evolved into a program that, the couple claims, has helped hundreds of thousands of people reach their weight-loss goals.

The Promise

Basic principles of Choose to Lose

According to the Goors, the primary cause of weight gain is not carbohydrates or even total calories, but dietary fat. By limiting fatty foods and filling up on the nutrient-dense, fiber-rich carbohydrate in fruit, vegetables, and whole grains, they maintain, you can easily and effectively shed the pounds that plague you—with the added bonus of improving your overall health

The explanation

Your body burns a certain amount of energy so that your heart, lungs, brain, and other major organs can function. This is your basal metabolic rate (BMR), also sometimes called your resting metabolic rate. Add to your BMR the energy burned during physical activity throughout the day, and you get the total amount of energy expended during that period. Where does energy come from? You take in energy with every morsel of food that passes your lips.

Of the three macronutrients—fat, protein, and carbohydrate—fat is the most densely packed with calories: It has nine calories per gram, while proteins and carbs have only four calories per gram. Not only do you consume a dense concentration of calories when you eat fat but, the Goors contend, the fat you eat is quickly stored, unlike protein and carbohydrate, which are rapidly burned off when eaten in reasonable amounts. The authors say that dietary fat is only utilized if your body needs more energy than it gets from protein and carbohydrate. The key to weight loss, they claim, is to eat less fat than you require to satisfy your energy needs; your body will make up for the deficit by mobilizing fat from its fat stores. Your "fat budget," as the Goors call it, is the maximum number of calories you're allowed to spend on fat each day and still lose weight safely. The authors provide charts and tables for calculating your fat budget, based on your height, frame size, and weight goals. For example, if you are a woman with a goal weight of 120 pounds, your fat budget is 281 fat calories a day.

> The key to weight loss, the Goors claim, is to eat less fat than you require to satisfy your energy needs.

One extremely important reason that the Goors emphasize reducing fat calories, not overall calories: They maintain that a diet too low in overall calories for your energy requirements will actually slow down weight loss because your body, in starvation mode, will reduce its BMR to conserve energy, and any dietary fat will continue to add weight. So, they claim, you need to have a reasonable overall caloric intake to keep your BMR cranking enough to burn fat.

Many popular diets hold that carbs—not dietary fat—pile on the pounds (see reviews of the Atkins diet, *Protein Power*, *The Carbohydrate Addict's Lifespan Program*, and *Sugar Busters!*). No way, say the Goors: You'd have to eat 2,200 calories of pure carbs a day above and beyond your normal caloric intake for five or six consecutive days to store carbohydrate as fat rather than use it as energy. In fact, they say, it's nearly impossible to overeat carbs, provided they're the right kind. The good carbs are vegetables, fruit, and whole grains, which, they say, make you feel full long before you've eaten too many calories. The authors do warn, however, that you can sabotage your weight-loss effort with so-called empty carbohydrate calories, such as from fat-free products and fiberless, nutrient-poor processed foods; these foods give you calories *without* making you feel full, so it's much easier to eat too much of them. And with excess carbohydrate calories at its disposal, the body doesn't get around to burning fat.

Evidence claimed

To support their approach, the Goors point more to the health effects of their diet than to specific evidence that it reduces weight. To back up their contention that a high-fat diet poses serious health risks, the Goors refer to a study in which men and women with normal cholesterol levels were fed high-fat and nonfat meals. The negative effects of the high-fat meal were immediately evident. Afterwards, oxidized, triglyceride-rich lipoproteins formed. This reaction, say the Goors, is a harbinger of atherosclerosis.

The health risks of a high-fat diet, the Goors claim, are evident if you look at what has been happening in Japan since fast-food restaurants were introduced there. In recent years that country, once renowned for its slender population and extremely low rate of heart disease, has experienced a precipitous rise in the incidence of obesity and heart disease. Not surprising, say the Goors, when you consider that a typical fast-food cheeseburger can have as many as 570 fat calories—a figure well over their recommendation of a daily fat budget for an average person.

The Method

How the Choose to Lose approach works

On the "choose to lose" program you eat three meals a day that have enough calories to meet your energy requirements, and that keep within your established fat budget. The authors provide one week of meal plans centered around low-fat, fiber-rich foods that, they say, will "keep your BMR chugging at its maximum rate" so that you have the best chance of burning stored fat. The Goors recommend that you follow the guidelines of the USDA's Food Guide Pyramid, a widely available reference that emphasizes keeping dietary fat down. Your diet should consist mainly of carbohydrates, especially high-fiber whole grains, veggies, and fruits.

You can eat what you like as long as you stay within your fat budget. The authors do recommend, however, that you limit high-fat meat such as lamb, beef, and pork to occasional treats, and even then that you should build the meal around veggies and rice rather than making meat the centerpiece. Other suggestions: Eat chicken and turkey without the skin; avoid hot dogs and packaged deli meats; limit cheese but eat lots of low- and nonfat dairy products for the

You can eat what you like as long as you stay within your fat budget.

calcium they contain; if you must use oil, use monounsaturated olive or canola oil, not polyunsaturated or hydrogenated oils; avoid salads since they're usually just conduits for fatty dressing; eat bread, especially whole grain, as well as pasta, rice, potatoes (no butter or cream sauce), and high-fiber breakfast cereal. Sugar isn't the pound-packer people have made it out to be, say the Goors, but you don't want to eat too much of it. Go ahead and use real jelly or jam, they say, and eat hard candies in moderation— but watch out for sugar-loaded "low-fat" cookies, snack bars, candies, and ice cream.

The authors further suggest that you make gradual adjustments to your diet. Can you realistically eliminate a fat source, or eat it less often, or replace it with a low-fat substitute? Make lists of fatty foods that you can eliminate or substitute for right away. After several weeks or months of incorporating such changes into your eating habits, you ought to make new lists and try to cut out additional fat. The key is gradual change, the authors say. In the case of milk, for example, you can go from drinking whole milk to 2% milk to 1% and finally to skim.

What you'll notice

After about 12 weeks on their program, the Goors assure you, you'll lose your "fat tooth." Other claims: Your energy will dramatically increase and the nutrients you'll be eating will strengthen your immune system and make your skin glow, your hair shine, and your teeth, gums, and bones strong. As for the rate of weight loss, be patient, the Goors counsel. People lose fat at different rates. They don't recommend constantly weighing yourself, since other factors such as temporary water retention might mislead you. Instead, the authors say, you should measure your progress by how your clothes fit.

Additional steps to take

Keep a thorough, accurate food record, the Goors counsel, to ferret out the main sources of fat in your diet, to determine how many fat calories you're eating each day, and to ensure you're getting the proper number of servings from different food groups. List all the food you eat in a day and document the total calories as well as the fat calories. You won't have to keep a food record for the rest of your life, the Goors say—just until you're aware of what foods and food combinations will keep you within your fat budget.

You don't need to take supplements by the megadose, according to the authors, since you'll be getting vitamins, minerals, fiber, antioxidants, and other important nutrients from your balanced diet.

The Diet as Lifestyle

Staying the course

The Goors claim that on their program you never have to feel guilty or deprived if you fit in fatty treats when your fat budget allows. You have to save fat calories so you can afford to indulge, though; if you eat a treat without prepayment, you'll soon find yourself in fat debt. Spontaneous splurging isn't a crime in the "choose to lose" program. Regain control and move on, they advise, trying to balance your fat intake over the next few days to get back on budget.

The Goors' approach is a lifetime change. If, in the future, you begin to regain weight, don't panic. They suggest that in such circumstances you reassess your eating habits and resume your food log to see where fat has slipped back into your meals. Make the necessary changes and within a short time, they say, you'll be back at your desired weight.

Getting into gear

The more muscle you have, the higher your BMR, say the Goors, and thus the easier it is to burn dietary fat. To build and preserve muscle, then, you need to incorporate exercise into your weight-loss approach. The Goors recommend 30 minutes of walking each day, not at breakneck pace but nonstop. Activities such as bicycling, swimming, and rowing are also beneficial because they speed up your metabolism and energy expenditure, helping you burn calories. To reap the full benefits of exercise, the Goors advise, stretch every day and include strength training in your schedule every other day. "Strength training will help you remain independent, strong, and flexible as you age," they promise.

Evaluating the Diet

Cautions and concerns

Losing weight gradually is better for you than crash dieting, and the Goors propose a slow-mo regimen that should appeal to just about any weight-loss hopefuls. Two of the authors' recommendations are particularly helpful: easing rather than galloping into a low-fat regimen, which they say will prevent a sense of deprivation, and using the USDA Food Guide Pyramid as a guideline to get the full array of nutrients available from a varied, balanced diet—especially one rich in high-fiber vegetables, fruit, and whole grains.

This sensible, nonprescriptive approach to eating is more important than the reasoning behind it, some of which is questionable. Dr. Goor's training and experience with the National Institutes of Health would suggest that he knows what he's talking about when it comes to the effects of fat on the human body. However, he and his wife offer no detailed evidence for what appears to be the centerpiece of their argument—that dietary fat is more fattening than protein or carbs of equivalent calories because of the way it is metabolized. The authors go against the grain of established research in asserting that it's not the total number of calories you eat but the amount of fat that packs on pounds. Studies suggest that indeed it is total calorie—not total fat—intake that is responsible for the increase in obesity in America. People today are eating less fat that they were 50 years ago, but they're fatter. The reason? They're consuming several hundred more calories per day than in the 1950s, and they're exercising less.

Many scientists question the wisdom of making a low-fat diet into a lifelong habit, as the Goors recommend, so some caution is in order. When people go on an extremely low-fat, high-carb diet and they don't exercise, they tend not to lose weight; their triglycerides go up, and their HDL (the good cholesterol) goes down, which sets the stage for heart disease. However, a diet like the Goors' that derives between 20 and 25% of its calories from fat is low in fat but not extremely so, and many studies have demonstrated that such a regimen can in fact reverse heart disease. Just keep in mind that going overboard with the low-fat approach can be unhealthful.

You might want to ignore the authors' advice to avoid salads because they are "high-fat outlets." Salads can be a terrific source of vitamins, minerals, antioxidants and fiber, as long as you choose your ingredients wisely (easy on the bacon bits) and don't slather on high-fat dressing.

Quick fix or lasting results?

According to the Goors, theirs is a lifetime plan because it teaches good eating habits. Though you won't lose 40 pounds in three weeks, if you stick with the program, chances are you'll eventually achieve your weight goal.

Flexible or rigid?

Supposedly, you can eat anything you want on the Goor plan. Here's the catch: You've got to fit what you eat into your fat budget, and that can be tight. You're allowed to derive only about 20% of your daily calories from fat. It won't take much dietary fat to strain your budget.

Stumbling blocks

The real drawback to this diet is developing the stomach for it. Fat is one of life's pleasures. It gives food flavor, staying power, and texture—crispy, or smooth, or creamy. Depending on your tastebuds, you may or may not believe the Goors when they promise that you'll learn to love low-fat living.

The Goors urge you to cook your own meals from scratch rather than eating prepared meals. This way you'll avoid food that's shot up with fat, sodium, and artificial ingredients, they say. Being your own chef requires planning and time, not least to keep your kitchen stocked with the abundant supply of fresh produce for which this program calls. And making a habit of always cooking your own meals will deprive you of another of life's joys—eating out. While the Goors' is a health-wise diet, it could turn out to be not much fun.

Is it for you?

If you're serious about losing weight and keeping it off—and you can live on a reduced-fat diet forever, or most of the time—this regimen might be the one for you. With its emphasis on high-fiber grains, vegetables and fruits, it should provide you with the nutrients you'll need to fuel and maintain your body while enabling you to shed weight gradually. And if you have heart disease, the "choose to lose" approach may help you reverse it. Diehard fans of fat, however, should keep in mind that certain weight-loss plans with higher fat content than the Goors' have proven effective in helping to prevent or reverse heart disease, including the southern Mediterranean diet (see the review of *Low-Fat Lies*), which emphasizes a reduction of *saturated* fat while allowing moderate amounts of unsaturated fat. If you have high triglycerides, it might be a good idea to consume a diet slightly higher in monounsaturated fat than the Goors'.

If you hate to cook or you're an incurable restaurant-hopper, this diet's not for you. As for diabetics and others with insulin-related disorders, you'd be better off shopping for a lower-carb plan. Check with your doctor.

Resources

The details of the Goors' weight-loss program can be found in *Choose to Lose: A Food Lover's Guide to Permanent Weight Loss* (Houghton Mifflin, 1999). To read more about the program, log on to www.choicediets.com, or call 1-888-897-9360. You can reach the authors by snail mail at Choose to Lose, P.O. Box 2053, Rockville, MD 20847-2053.

The Diet Cure

Julia Ross attributes the struggles people have with weight, food cravings, and mood swings to biochemical imbalances and nutrient loss. As executive director of Recovery Systems, a clinic in California that treats eating disorders and weight problems, Ross claims to have seen firsthand how nutrient therapy and biochemical rebalancing, along with counseling and education, can bring quick relief to clients whose previous attempts to control weight left them dispirited. *The Diet Cure: The 8-Step Program to Rebalance Your Body Chemistry and End Food Cravings, Weight Problems, and Mood Swings—Now* explains her approach. Ross, who has a masters degree in clinical psychology, bases her program on 10 years of what she says are proven clinical results. She refers to her book as a repair manual that will help you "find and fix the physical malfunctions that have caused your particular eating, mood, weight, or health problems." In her hands, says Ross, you'll learn how to rebalance your body and feel better in a matter of days—perhaps even hours.

The Promise

Basic principles of the Diet Cure

Ross contends that many people with weight problems are heavy not because they lack self-control, but because their bodies are malfunctioning. Often the problem results from years of dieting, a harmful practice, says Ross, that depletes your system of vital nutrients and negatively affects your mood, energy level, and overall health. Junk food is another problem. Ross blames health problems associated with obesity not on fat but on too many "bad" carbohydrates in the American diet—primarily from refined-sugar products such as sweets and candies. Your body may be so damaged, says Ross, that diet alone cannot restore it to proper balance. Eating good food isn't enough to keep you healthy, she goes on, because factors such as light, heat, and inadequate soil can sap food of nutrients before it gets to your table. In addition to changing your eating habits, therefore, she recommends dietary supplements—lots of them.

Following Ross's recommendations, she makes clear, won't transform you into a skinny supermodel; rather, it will restore you to your natural weight. "It is your body's job to maintain its genetically programmed features, including its weight," she warns. "Try to alter that weight at your peril."

The explanation

According to Ross, there are eight physical conditions that may be triggering your specific problem: brain chemistry imbalance, low-calorie dieting, unstable blood sugar, low thyroid function, addiction to food you're allergic to, hormonal havoc, yeast overgrowth, and fatty acid deficiency. You may have one or more of these conditions, she says. For each one, she lists symptoms and maps out dietary changes to correct it.

Though Ross advocates taking vitamins and minerals, the key to her diet cure is amino acids, which are sold as supplements in health food stores. These protein fragments, says Ross, are the miracle foods used by your brain to manufacture "powerful pleasure chemicals," including serotonin, dopamine/norepinephrine, and endorphin. Ross contends that if you supplement your diet with the appropriate amino acids, your general mood will lift, anxiety will disappear, and once-powerful cravings for food, alcohol, and drugs will evaporate—usually within 24 hours of the first dose.

"It is your body's job to maintain its genetically programmed features, including its weight," Ross warns. "Try to alter that weight at your peril."

To support her claim about the dramatic effects of amino acids on addictive behavior, Ross refers to "hundreds of research studies at Harvard, MIT, and elsewhere" without, however, offering specific information. She does cite one particular study done at the University of Texas suggesting that people at the end of a diet regimen can avert weight regain by taking amino acids. And, she claims, 90% of the compulsive overeaters treated at her clinic with amino acids lost their addictions within 48 hours.

As for dietary supplements, Ross refers to a summary of data from "three major nationwide surveys" showing that "one of every two American women consumed inadequate amounts of almost every vitamin and mineral studied." She also mentions a study of 400 women published in the British Medical Journal demonstrating that multivitamin supplements reduced the risk of delivering babies with congenital abnormalities by 50%, as well as a study of 900 people over a 10-year period in which multivitamin supplements cut the risk of colon cancer by half.

Ross is not a doctor. To make you feel more at ease with her program, she includes a list of her board of advisors for the book—two medical doctors and two PhDs, all with expertise in some aspect of nutrition and/or neurochemistry. Much of the information in the book, however, is based on Ross's experience as director of the Recovery Center. When recommending doses of a particular supplement, she'll mention what dose tends to work best for most of her clients. On occasion she'll include a case study describing a single patient's quick response to treatment and ultimate success on the diet cure program.

The Method

How the Diet Cure works

The first step is to fill out Ross's "quick symptom questionnaire" and determine which of the eight physical imbalances plagues you. To see if you are addicted to foods you're allergic to, for instance, you score yourself on cravings for specific foods, family history of food allergies, and digestive discomforts after eating certain foods. After identifying your problem, you consult Ross's recommendations for dietary changes and create a "master plan" for yourself. If you want, you can craft your plan in consultation with a qualified professional such as a nutritionist or dietician.

The approach varies depending on what Ross says ails you, whether it's "depleted brain chemistry," a low-calorie diet, a thyroid problem, or something else. Regardless of your specific ailment, however, there are certain guidelines that Ross advises everyone on her plan to follow. For example, she supports the USDA's standards of minimum calories per day: 2,500 for women and 2,800 for men—numbers that vary somewhat with your height and activity level. What you eat to fulfill that calorie requirement, she contends, is crucial. For good nutrition, says Ross, you need a minimum of four cups of vegetables a day, fruit, protein—adults should have at least 20 grams at each meal, whether it's fish, beans, eggs, lean meat, chicken, or tofu—and "good" carbohydrates such as those found in vegetables, beans, and whole grains. Eat organic food whenever that's possible, counsels Ross, and you'll be reducing your intake of pesticides, antibiotics, and growth hormones. She advises that about a third of your total calories come from the fat found in avocados, nuts, seeds, and fish, though butter is allowed; this will keep you feeling satisfied so you don't overeat junk food in search of satisfaction, Ross says. Avoid hydrogenated fats, she cautions, because they've been linked to heart disease, cancer, and arthritis. Cut out sugar, sugar substitutes, fried foods, processed meat, caffeinated and carbonated beverages, and even iceberg lettuce, which she claims contributes to constipation and other intestinal problems. Keep your ratio of carb to

Ross promises that if you eat foods that make you feel strong and energetic, you'll be healthy—and you won't have to count calories or fat grams religiously.

protein at about two to one (you can measure by grams or calories), she counsels, and whatever you do, don't skip meals.

Ross promises that if you eat foods that make you feel strong and energetic, you'll be healthy—and you won't have to count calories or fat grams religiously. To get you eating healthfully, Ross includes a list of foods rich in nutrients, a two-week menu plan, and a selection of recipes, among them protein smoothies, lemon-scented rice salad, turkey burgers, and creamy polenta.

What you'll notice

Lots of changes occur during the first week of her plan, Ross claims. Within 24 hours of beginning supplements, she says, clients consistently find that their mood lifts and their cravings disappear. By day five, your food cravings are supposed to vanish entirely. Ross warns that you may lose your appetite or feel queasy the first four days. If nausea continues for more than two days, it might be the supplements that are bothering you. Stop them, she counsels, and add them back one at a time to identify the culprits. If you experience other withdrawal symptoms, such as weariness and headaches, over-the-counter painkillers will help. In the first week, she adds, you also may lose more weight than at any other point—perhaps up to seven pounds—especially if you're renouncing foods you're allergic to.

When you reach week four, Ross warns, you may struggle with afternoon or evening cravings. Typically this is because you aren't eating enough nutritious food. Add more protein, fat, or whole-grain carbs to your meals, she suggests.

Over the months, says Ross, as your body moves toward biochemical balance, you'll slowly and steadily acquire your natural, ideal shape and weight. The process should be completed, she adds, within three to 12 months.

Additional steps to take

Ross recommends a multivitamin and mineral supplement to replenish your body's nutrients and maintain them, along with additional doses of magnesium and calcium, a basic B complex vitamin, vitamin C with bioflavonoids, vitamin E, fish oil, and chromium. According to the author, you may also need to take special "repair" supplements such as amino acids, St. John's Wort, or zinc to correct any of the eight imbalances you might have. These supplements can be stopped as soon as your problem resolves itself.

It's extremely important, says Ross, to listen to your body's signals about the foods and supplements you give it. She recommends keeping a detailed "food-mood log" that records everything you've ingested and when. Did you eat the recommended amount of protein at each meal? What was your protein-to-carb ratio? How about vegetables? Supplements? If you have cravings during the day, write them down and state when they occur. Record how you feel throughout the day, both emotionally and physically, and note how well you slept the night before. Write down what kind of exercise you've done that day and comment on how you felt before and after. Keep the log daily for a few months, Ross advises. Once you've learned to listen to the messages your body is sending, you can limit the log to problem days.

You may need to have blood, urine, and other medical tests done to determine what biochemical imbalances or other medical conditions you have, says Ross. She urges you to choose a doctor who will be open to the philosophy behind her program.

The Diet as Lifestyle

Staying the course

Ross claims that if you find yourself eating unhealthy foods after starting her program, you'll notice that you don't need as much of them as you once did to feel satisfied. However, she warns, if you stray too far you'll throw your biochemical balance off and be back at square one. If that happens, there's no need to chastise yourself or drown your sorrows in a junk-food binge. Instead, she advises, examine what pushed you off the plan. Often there's a logical explanation, such as skipping a meal or undereating.

After three to 12 months, Ross says, your body will be permanently balanced and you'll no longer need corrective supplements, though you should continue taking vitamin and mineral pills.

Getting into gear

Don't feel guilty if you're not exercising enough right now, says Ross. People beset with imbalances have little energy for physical activity. When your body is balanced, you'll have more energy and you'll want to exercise regularly, Ross maintains. She advocates strengthening exercise, stretching, and aerobics. You need some form of aerobic exercise at least four times a week for a minimum of 15 to 20 minutes, according to Ross. Choose an activity you enjoy.

Beware of becoming an exercise addict, warns Ross. If you feel anxious when you can't get to the gym every day, you might be relying on exercise to counteract a biochemical imbalance. If you exercise a lot but have no energy, she says, you might have exhausted your adrenal glands, in which case exercise is sapping you of the little energy you can muster.

Ross also strongly recommends relaxation techniques, which, she says, will enhance your results on her plan and help lengthen your life. She gives a long list of relaxation tips, including periodic breaks during the day, plenty of sleep at night, and regular vacations.

Evaluating the Diet

Cautions and concerns

Ross's dietary recommendations—consuming whole grains, beans, nuts, fish, and an abundance of fresh produce; meeting your fat needs by sticking mostly to unsaturated sources; and cutting out sugary and processed junk food—will contribute to healthy eating. Nonetheless, her program should be approached cautiously by would-be weight losers. It is unlikely that you'll crunch pounds on a diet of 2,500 calories for women or 2,800 calories for men. According to Ross, it's what you eat that puts on padding. "Bad" carbs, she announces, are the cause of American obesity. In fact, people gain weight by consuming too many calories whether they eat well-balanced diets or subsist on soda and doughnuts. To cast off the pounds that calorie-loading has stuck you with, you'll probably have to consume a diet lower in calories than Ross's program.

While Ross's general food recommendations are nutritionally sound, the science underpinning her plan isn't reliable. Ross is not a trained physician, and her theory attributing excess weight, mood swings, food cravings, and addictions to eight biochemical "imbalances" oversimplifies the complex machinery of the human body. What, for example, does a food craving signal? A biochemical imbalance, as Ross would have it? A certain nutrient in the coveted food that your body needs? Or some other condition? Changing your diet according to Ross's prescription may not spell the cure. "There are such enormous psychosocial effects on appetite that it's hard to separate out changes caused by what's in the diet," says endocrinologist Gerald Reaven of Stanford University.

Ross's so-called diet cure program relies heavily on supplements. Vitamins and minerals taken in excessive doses or in combination with certain medicines or medical conditions can be toxic. Most mainstream nutritionists, while they don't discourage taking a multivitamin/mineral supplement, recommend that people derive the bulk of their vitamin and mineral needs from a balanced, varied diet. At any rate, there is little evidence to support Ross's various claims that certain supplements will cure specific biochemical imbalances. As for amino acids being "miracle foods" that will lift your mood, abolish anxiety, and eradicate cravings for food, alcohol and drugs, her claims are unsubstantiated.

Quick fix or lasting results?

A diet that recommends as many calories as this one is unlikely to result in weight loss, either in the short or in the long term.

Flexible or rigid?

No rigorous counting of calories or fat grams on this one. And while Ross recommends a ratio of 2 to 1 carbs to protein, she urges you to find the ratio that works best for you. Though the author's dietary restrictions make good nutritional sense, some people might find them a tad puritanical—no caffeine, no soda, no sugar or sugar substitutes, no fried foods.

Stumbling blocks

You may be sorely taxed sorting through all the information about ailments and how to cure them with specific supplement combinations and dosages. Once you've puzzled out your master plan, you'll be popping pills and capsules throughout the day—so many that Ross recommends you "lay out your supplements in either small labeled plastic bags or plastic boxes with dividers." She also suggests an alarm or pager so that you're reminded to take supplements between meals. All this could put a hefty dent in your wallet—and complicate life for the hectic traveler. One other drawback for busy folks: You'll have to squeeze enough time from the day to fill out your "food-mood log."

Is it for you?

If you truly do have hormone problems, insulin-related disorders, allergies, excessive mood swings, or other potentially serious medical conditions, you'd do well to consult a qualified health-care professional before choosing an entrée in Ross's menu of remedies—a step the author herself recommends. It's also not a bad idea to consult a physician before launching a supplementation plan that goes above and beyond the government's recommended daily requirements. People with an incurable sweet tooth won't survive long on this chuck-the-sugar plan. And if your hope is to shed pounds in a jiffy, Ross's high-calorie plan probably won't support your goal. If, however, you'd like to cast aside crutches such as sugar and caffeine and be steered away from junk food toward nature's fresh, organic bounty, then Ross may be the guide you've been seeking. Take her basic dietary recommendations, subtract 1,000 calories from the daily calorie allotment, and you'll probably end up losing weight—the health-wise way.

Resources

You can learn the nuts and bolts of Ross's program by obtaining a copy of *The Diet Cure: The 8-Step Program to Rebalance Your Body Chemistry and End Food Cravings, Weight Problems, and Mood Swings—Now* (Viking 1999) and visiting the author's website at www.dietcure.com. The book will tell you how to contact counselors, nutritionists, holistic doctors, and other health professionals. You can write Julia Ross at The Diet Cure, 775 E. Blithedale #402, Mill Valley, CA 94941. To speak with someone at the Recovery Systems Clinic, call 415-458-8466.

Dieting with the Duchess: Secrets and Sensible Advice for a Great Body

Sarah, Duchess of York and former wife of Britain's Prince Andrew, teamed up with Weight Watchers to offer this book of guidelines for successful weight control. A spokesperson for Weight Watchers International, she shares lessons from her real-life weight-loss struggles and touts the benefits of Weight Watchers' 1·2·3 Success® plan. The diet she espouses, based on balance, variety, and moderation, follows the general recommendations of the USDA Food Guide Pyramid. Sarah rejects the quick-fix claims of fad diets, advocating instead a long-term change in lifestyle that promotes good health as it slowly but steadily helps you reach and maintain your ideal body weight.

The Promise

Basic principles

Sarah enlarges on the Weight Watchers philosophy of weight control with advice about exercise and how to handle the emotional issues that can make or break a weight-loss campaign. In essence, Weight Watchers promotes a low-calorie, low-fat, high-fiber diet using a point system. Foods are assigned a point value based on calories, fat, and fiber content. You're allotted a specific range of total points each day, typically 22 to 29 points—depending on your current body weight and your weight goal—which you can "spend" however you like. (See the review of the Weight Watchers plan.)

But to lose weight, says Sarah, you shouldn't be on a diet per se. The changes you make to rein in your weight are really lifestyle changes. Sarah presents herself as a role model with whom you can identify—a duchess, but also a vulnerable woman. If you follow the tenets of the lifestyle she describes, you'll peel off pounds just as she did, says Sarah. And you'll control your weight for the long haul.

The explanation

Many diet gurus would have you believe that some calories count less than others in the battle of the bulge. Hold on, says Sarah: Every calorie you put in your mouth can affect your weight. "No matter who you are, if you consume more calories than you expend, you'll gain weight; if you burn more calories than you consume, you'll lose weight." This doesn't mean you have to renounce the foods you love in order to shed unwanted pounds. No foods have to be taboo, she maintains, as long as you monitor your portions, eat a varied and balanced diet, and exercise regularly: "The key to healthful eating is to make savvy choices from the Food Guide Pyramid and balance your favorite foods with those that promote good health."

"No matter who you are, if you consume more calories than you expend, you'll gain weight; if you burn more calories than you consume, you'll lose weight."

The Food Guide Pyramid advocates six to 11 servings daily of grain foods, three to five servings of vegetables, two to four servings of fruit, two to three servings of milk, yogurt and cheese, two to three servings of meat, poultry, fish, beans, eggs, and nuts, and sparing use of fats and sweets. Weight Watchers' 1·2·3 Success plan follows the pyramid. Carefully monitor your portion sizes to make sure you aren't overeating, Sarah advises. Since clinical trials have shown that increasing the amount of fruits and vegetables in a diet lowers the risk of some cancers, you should give these foods a starring role. Dairy products, especially milk fortified with calcium and vitamin D, are also important, but choose low-fat or skim varieties to avoid excessive fat.

Evidence claimed

To support her weight-loss principles, Sarah refers to the National Weight Control Registry, an ongoing project that so far has tracked the progress of 2,800 people who've lost at least 30 pounds and kept it off for more than a year. This is the largest study to date on successful weight losers and their weight-management techniques. Each of the dieters tried and failed to keep weight off before adopting successful strategies. What made them finally shed weight and sustain the loss, says Sarah, was sticking to a low-fat, low-calorie diet and exercising regularly. They also limited their intake of certain high-fat foods and controlled their portions. Most ate several small meals throughout the day (five meals on average, including snacks) and tended not to eat out.

References to various other studies support specific points about the behavior of dieters and the medical importance of including certain foods in the diet. But the bulk of the evidence Sarah musters lies in her personal testimony. What worked for her was abiding by the general recommendations of the Food Guide Pyramid (especially limiting dietary fat) and eating food in moderation. There are no figures stating how many people have followed her approach—or the Weight Watchers plan she endorses—and lost weight. Nor does she say exactly how much weight she has lost.

The Method

How it works

Sarah starts you on a four-week eating plan tailored for weight loss of up to two pounds a week. The menus, simple but not repetitive, get you on track with the Weight Watchers approach without making you agonize over portions. Each menu carries a Weight Watchers point value.

Once you've completed the initial phase you're ready to create your own meal plans. Sarah offers tips on balanced, nutritious cuisine. Some 50% of the day's calories should come from carbohydrates (mostly complex carbs such as beans and whole grains), about 20% from protein, and no more than 30% from fats. Make sure you include 20 to 30 grams of fiber each day, but if you're currently eating much less, work up to that goal slowly. Fiber promotes a healthy digestive tract and has the added benefit of making you feel full longer on fewer calories. Most Americans eat much more protein than they need (sometimes twice as much). Sarah recommends that you monitor your intake and select low-fat sources such as nonfat yogurt and white-fleshed fish instead of red meat. Fat should be eaten in moderation and mainly in monounsaturated form, for example, olive oil.

What you'll notice

According to the National Weight Control Registry study cited by Sarah, 85% of the participants said that after losing 30 pounds they had more energy and more self-confidence. Most found that their health and general mood improved, as did their relationships, even with strangers. Sarah assures you that you, too, will feel more confident and energetic, and less fatigued, after adopting a healthy lifestyle.

Additional steps to take

If you want to monitor what you're eating, particularly your fat intake, you need to make a habit of reading food labels, says Sarah. And since dieters are at special risk of not getting all the vitamins and minerals they need, it's smart to take a multivitamin supplement as a precaution. Drink plenty of water, at least six 8-ounce glasses a day, to carry waste products from your body, help with digestion, control your body temperature, and lubricate your joints.

Sarah also recommends that you cultivate your self-esteem. Learn to accept and value yourself as you are now, she urges, before you begin to lose weight. In other words, "strive to be the best person you can be," and don't try to "look like some cultural ideal." Weight Watchers' Tools for Living, a set of techniques for coping with the thoughts and feelings that threaten to lay waste to your weight-loss plans, can help, Sarah maintains. Techniques include "reframing," a way of replacing negative behavior with positive, and mental rehearsing, in which you envision yourself saying no to temptation.

Research, says Sarah, has shown that keeping a food diary, an exercise log, and a mood journal are all effective aids when you're trying to alter your lifestyle. They record your progress and your slip-ups, holding you accountable for your actions and reinforcing your commitment to change.

The Diet as Lifestyle

Staying the course

It's typical to have setbacks—major and minor—when you're making lifestyle changes. Don't waste time flagellating yourself for stumbling; forgive and move on. If you're on the verge of bingeing, do something enjoyable to distract yourself, such as taking a walk, reading a book, or playing with your kids.

So as not to overwhelm yourself by dramatic change, take things day by day. "If you begin every morning with the idea that you have a fresh opportunity to eat more healthfully, to pack in plenty of exercise, and to begin to peel off excess pounds, you'll stay more motivated," says Sarah. End each day by patting yourself on the back for all the things you did well, not kicking yourself for things you might have done better. You'll need that kind of motivation, she warns, because maintaining weight loss is a lifetime commitment. Even after reaching your weight goal you'll have to monitor yourself, managing the balancing act of counting calories and fat grams without becoming obsessed with your diet.

Getting into gear

E xercise is critical in the effort to trim fat and keep it off. Sarah follows the U.S. Surgeon General's recommendation of 30 minutes of physical activity—either all at once or broken up—most days of the week. She advocates aerobic exercise, strength training, and flexibility exercises. The key to making exercise a part of your daily life, says Sarah, is to choose workouts you enjoy. Cross-training will keep you from getting bored. What are the payoffs of exercise? Studies have shown that regular exercise increases the chances of a longer, healthier life. Exercise, claims Sarah, boosts your immune system; helps you sleep better; reduces your risk of cancer, heart disease, and osteoporosis; heats up your sex life; improves your mood and mental acuity; and enhances your body image. Schedule exercise into your calendar as if it's a business appointment, Sarah suggests, and keep an exercise journal to document your commitment. The Weight Watchers Activity Plan can help you set up and stick with an exercise program.

> The key to making exercise a part of your daily life, says Sarah, is to choose workouts you enjoy.

Evaluating the Diet

Cautions and concerns

S arah's suggestions, founded on the principle of choice bounded by balance, variety, and moderation, echo the approach of the USDA Food Guide Pyramid and Weight Watchers. There's nothing outlandish here: a moderately low-fat, low-calorie, high-fiber diet rich in vegetables and fruit, with no banned foods. But Sarah's message is a tad confusing. You shouldn't be dieting to lose weight, she says—you should be eating more healthfully, exercising, and watching portions. The plan she generally espouses, though, is a weight-loss diet, one that ranges roughly from 1,200 to 1,700 calories a day depending on your weight and other factors. The idea is to reduce caloric intake without outlawing the foods you love, but also to eat a variety of balanced, nutritious foods; the question is, how do you gain balance and still eat the cheeseburger and chocolate mousse you'd die for? Unless you're vigilant about monitoring the make-up of your meals, the leeway Sarah allows in food choices may cause you to fall short of your nutritional requirements— or gain weight.

Quick fix or lasting results?

Patience is a virtue in this program. Although Sarah doesn't say how long she's been practicing what she preaches, she does mention that at the time her book was published she'd been following her approach for two years. Because it takes years to establish unhealthful eating habits and turn fat, she warns, you need to give yourself plenty of time to break those habits. To lose weight, says Sarah, you shouldn't be on a crash diet: You should practice a lifetime regimen of exercise, portion control, and sensible food choices, always keeping the big picture in mind.

Flexible or rigid?

With no forbidden foods and no stipulations about when to eat or how often, this is a relatively flexible program despite the requirements of balanced nutrition. You can splurge occasionally, as long as you plan ahead and adjust other meals that day to compensate.

Stumbling blocks

Unlike Weight Watchers, Sarah doesn't recommend specific calorie counts to guide you in your weight-loss effort, nor does she suggest how to determine your weight goal. It's up to you to count calories, measure portions, and set goals. Up to you, also, to keep a food diary as well as exercise and mood journals. Dieters hard-pressed for time might find all this a tall order. After all, they'll be busy planning meals and learning new recipes as they strive to get more variety into their diets.

Is the Duchess of York really the right role model to inspire busy, weight-challenged women? While Sarah tries to portray herself as a single working mother just like you, she admits that she has a cook and a personal trainer. Chances are she's not making frenzied trips to the grocery store on her way home from work.

Is it for you?

Sarah's diet, which bans no foods but stresses healthy choices and exercise, reflects the sort of kinder, gentler approach to weight loss that has proven successful for many overweight people. The National Weight Control Registry offers good evidence for this approach. The database tracks people who have lost 30 pounds or more and kept them off for at least a year. Of its 2,800 participants, more than half accomplished their goals not by torturing themselves on a joyless diet, but by cutting down on fat, focusing on an overall healthy approach to eating—and exercising. If you have the nutritional know-how, discipline, and creativity to overhaul your lifestyle, this diet might be just what the doctor ordered.

If, however, you want closer guidance and a support group, your best bet is to join Weight Watchers. While Sarah doesn't overtly promote this group, she encourages you to participate in its 1·2·3 Success plan. Her list of 75 recipes and her four-week meal plan include 1·2·3 Success point values.

Sarah strives to identify with the reader by presenting herself as a working mother who suffers from lapses in self-esteem. Men, shop elsewhere.

Resources

Read all about this approach in *Dieting with the Duchess: Secrets and Sensible Advice for a Great Body* (Simon and Schuster, 1998), which the Duchess co-authored with Weight Watchers. To learn more about the Weight Watchers program, call 800-651-6000 or log on to www.weightwatchers.com. If you're looking for more recipes with Sarah's stamp of approval, pick up a copy of *Dining with Sarah: Making Everyday Meals a Special Occasion* (Simon and Schuster, 1998).

Eat More, Weigh Less

Dean Ornish, M.D., author of *Eat More, Weigh Less: Dr. Dean Ornish's Life Choice Program for Losing Weight Safely While Eating Abundantly*, developed his weight-loss program after doing groundbreaking research in the reversal of heart disease. The key elements of his regimen, which emphasizes health and well-being as well as weight loss, are a very-low-fat vegetarian diet, regular exercise, and stress management. In addition to being the author of several best-selling diet and health books, Ornish is founder and director of the nonprofit Preventive Medicine Research Institute in Sausalito, California. He teaches medicine at the University of California, San Francisco, where he established the Osher Center for Integrative Medicine. His message? Cut dietary fat to less than 10% of your total calories and you'll lose weight.

The Promise

Basic principles of the Ornish program

Most Americans consume around 40% of their calories as fat, Ornish claims. If you want to lose weight, he maintains, you should cut your fat intake to less than 10%. His so-called Life Choice diet works, he says, because it involves this dramatic reduction in dietary fat. How is it possible to slash fat intake? By focusing on the type of food you eat rather than the amount, the author says. You don't have to count calories or measure food portions. Instead, he says, you should eat foods that are very low in fat and high in complex carbohydrates and fiber. That means avoiding most animal foods, which come bundled with fat and contain little fiber, and concentrating instead on beans and other legumes, grains, fruits, and vegetables.

Ornish believes that going on a low-fat high-carb diet is the only way to avoid the dieter's curse: rollercoaster weight loss and regain. Why? Because, he claims, your metabolism doesn't slow down when you eat lots of carbohydrate and little fat, as it does on conventional calorie-restrictive diets.

The explanation

A gram of dietary fat has more than twice as many calories as a gram of either protein or carbohydrate. It's also more likely to be converted into body fat, says Ornish. On his very-low-fat diet, he promises, you can eat the same amount of food as before and you'll watch your waistline shrink.

Ornish argues that your metabolism—the rate at which your body expends energy—stays the same or increases on his Life Choice diet. This distinguishes his program, he says, from conventional calorie-restrictive diets that slow down the metabolism to compensate for the drop in calories. It's this slowing down of metabolism that's responsible for the weight "plateau" that many dieters experience after shedding a few pounds. How does Ornish's diet keep your body burning calories at a faster clip? When you eat a high-carb low-fat diet, he claims, your body converts more of the thyroid hormone thyroxin into an active form that spurs your metabolism on.

Another advantage of his program, says Ornish, is that you eat foods like whole grains and legumes that make you feel full before you've devoured too many calories. His diet is rich in fiber, which slows down the absorption of nutrients and staves off hunger pangs for longer periods. Blood sugar levels also remain more constant, and that, he claims, imparts a sense of well-being and equanimity.

Evidence claimed

According to Ornish, evolution has not caught up with modern American eating habits. Our bodies are designed, he says, for a world of scarcity; in times of food shortage, body fat is our backup fuel. Putting on weight easily gave our ancestors an evolutionary advantage—what Ornish calls "survival of the fattest." But food scarcity is no longer a problem for most Americans. That fact, coupled with our more sedentary lives, has made us a lot pudgier than our forebears. Ornish attributes America's current weight problem not to mere calories but to an overconsumption of fat. He cites statistics showing that Americans actually take in fewer calories today than they did 100 years ago, but that the proportion of calories we get from fatty foods has doubled.

> Putting on weight easily gave our ancestors an evolutionary advantage—what Ornish calls "survival of the fattest."

Ornish supports his low-fat high-carb approach by citing studies of his own. Since 1977, the author has been researching how to prevent and reverse heart disease. His studies, called collectively the Lifestyle Heart Trial, show that his recommended lifestyle changes can help reverse heart disease without drugs or surgery. The 22 patients in his trial experienced an average cholesterol drop of 40%, says Ornish. He also claims that participants in the first study lost an average of 22 pounds, even though they ate more food and more frequently.

Ornish also cites numerous studies besides his own to support his position. According to Ornish, one Cornell University study found that women on a low-fat diet lost twice as much weight as women on a calorie-restricted diet. Another study from Stanford University compared the diets of fat and thin men and found that although both groups consumed the same number of calories, the overweight men ate more fat. Ornish also notes that the average person in China gets 30% more total calories than the average American yet weighs less. The reason, he claims, is that the Chinese get 60% fewer calories from fat than Americans.

"Living leaner may help you live longer," Ornish says. For support, he cites animal studies. One compared the longevity of mice on a calorie-restricted high-fat diet, a calorie-restricted low-fat diet, and a diet of unlimited food. Mice on the calorie-restricted high-fat diet lived twice as long as mice given an unlimited amount of food—an impressive result. But mice on the calorie-restricted low-fat diet lived three times longer. Ornish concludes that although any kind of calorie restriction may help lengthen your life, your best bet is to restrict fat calories.

The Method

How the Ornish program works

The Life Choice diet, says Ornish, is not strictly speaking a diet "but rather a new way of eating." Ornish argues that it's important—and easiest—to switch to his radical diet all at once, so his plan has no stages. If you do it gradually, he says, the changes in your weight and well-being won't be dramatic enough to motivate you to let go of your favorite foods. Ornish does acknowledge, however, that switching to a low-fat vegetarian diet can be difficult and advises his readers to follow the program for at least two weeks before deciding whether or not it's working for them.

You can eat beans and other legumes, fruits, grains, and vegetables whenever you're hungry, Ornish assures you. Just be sure to stop eating when you feel full—don't stuff yourself. You're also allowed a moderate intake of nonfat dairy products, nonfat mayonnaise and salad dressings, and other nonfat or very-low-fat commercial foods such as whole-wheat breakfast cereal. He also touts his own brand of Life Choice frozen dinners.

Foods to avoid on the Ornish plan? Meat, chicken, and fish; all kinds of oil, including olive oil; oil-containing margarine and salad dressings; sugar and simple sugar derivatives, including honey and molasses; alcohol; avocados; olives; nuts, and seeds; high- and low-fat dairy products (the low-fat products are not that low in fat, he points out—stick with nonfat dairy); egg yolks; and any commercial foods that contain more than two grams of fat per serving.

Ornish urges you to plan quiet, leisurely meals and avoid double-tasking at mealtimes—gulping down your food while watching television or reading the newspaper, for example. Eat slowly, he says, and savor each bite. Your brain takes about 20 minutes to register that you're full, he adds, so the more slowly you eat, the less likely you are to overeat.

What you'll notice

During the first week on the Life Choice diet, you should lose weight, gain energy, and experience a greater sense of well-being, says Ornish. He also claims that you'll experience a drop in blood pressure and significantly lower cholesterol levels. If you have heart disease that causes angina, Ornish adds, chances are you'll notice a drastic reduction in the frequency of chest pains within a few days to a few weeks of going on his diet.

You'll also notice changes in your tastebuds, says Ornish. Fat, he argues, is an acquired taste. He says you'll soon adjust, for example, to the more watery taste of skim (nonfat) milk; after a few weeks milk with any degree of fat will taste too rich, like cream. You'll have a similar negative reaction to other fatty foods, he adds.

Additional steps to take

Reducing stress is another essential element of Ornish's program. He recommends spending an hour a day practicing techniques such as stretching, breathing, prayer, progressive relaxation, and especially meditation, which he dubs "food for your soul."

In addition, on his official website (see Resources) Ornish recommends vitamin and mineral supplements. He suggests a daily multivitamin without iron for men and post-menopausal women. (Premenopausal women may benefit from iron supplements, he says, but others should avoid them because iron creates free radicals, molecules that can damage your cells and hasten aging.) Other daily supplements: vitamin C, vitamin E, folic acid, selenium, and fish oil. To these supplements women should add flaxseed oil, says Ornish. He does not recommend flaxseed oil for men because of evidence he cites that links it to the growth of prostate cancer cells.

The Diet as Lifestyle

Staying the course

According to Ornish, eating with "awareness" rather than mindlessly shoveling in the food will help you stick with his program. Reaching out to others for emotional support can fortify you as well. Support groups, he claims, are "a powerful factor in helping you to lose weight and to keep it off." According to Ornish, they can also prolong your life. "People who feel socially isolated have two to five times the incidence of disease and premature death due to all causes as those who feel a sense of community and connection," he says. So he recommends joining a diet support group that meets once or twice a week.

Getting into gear

On his diet, Ornish says, you won't need to burn off as many fat calories as on a typical calorie-restrictive diet. Still, he recommends regular moderate exercise. A 30- to 60-minute daily walk is often enough, he says. He points to studies suggesting that moderate exercise may actually be better at helping you lose weight than intensive exercise such as "power" walking or running. Researchers, he claims, have found that during short, intense exercise the body tends to burn carbohydrates as fuel, while during longer, slower activity it burns fat. Moderate exercise also tends to subdue the appetite, says Ornish, while intense exercise can cause you to make a beeline for the refrigerator.

Ornish recommends combining aerobic exercise with moderate resistance training, such as light weight lifting, rowing, or stair climbing. Resistance training builds muscle, which can speed up your metabolism permanently, he says.

Evaluating the Diet

Cautions and concerns

It's true that eating high-fiber, low-calorie-dense foods such as beans, other legumes, fruits, and vegetables will fill you up with fewer calories than fatty foods deliver. It's also true that these foods are good for you. But so are some of the foods that Ornish disapproves of, such as fish and low-fat dairy products.

Ornish's plan has been proven effective in significantly lowering LDL—the "bad" cholesterol that can build plaque in arteries and lead to heart disease. But there are some reasons to question whether a severe low-fat program such as this is the ideal diet for overweight people in general, or even for those with heart disease. The diet Ornish had his patients follow in the Lifestyle Heart Trial did not lower triglycerides (blood fat), for example, and it failed to raise HDL, the "good" cholesterol. This effect on cholesterol levels is commonly seen in people who follow low-fat high-carb diets, suggesting that such regimens would possibly increase the risk of heart disease. As for the cardiac benefits that Ornish's study did demonstrate, it isn't clear how closely linked they were to the diet itself, since patients simultaneously engaged in exercise and other stress-reducing practices such as meditation, which can improve the condition of heart disease patients.

What Ornish doesn't mention is the famous Lyon Heart Study in France, which showed a dramatic reduction in cardiac disease symptoms—comparable to the reduction seen in Ornish's own group—among patients following a Mediterranean-style diet rich in olive and canola oil, both monounsaturated fats. The Lyon Heart Study followed 300 patients as opposed to Ornish's 22, and it controlled its variables, with patients following a specific diet but not engaging in a special exercise or meditation regimen. (See the review of *Low-Fat Lies*.)

Ornish takes a blanket stance against dietary fat. But olive oil, a monounsaturated fat, has been shown to improve cholesterol levels by slightly hiking HDL levels and slightly lowering LDL and triglycerides. In other words, olive oil can be heart-healthy. Studies show that limiting saturated fat is more important than limiting total fat in reducing blood cholesterol levels—and that cutting fat intake to just 27% of total calories can help reduce the risk of heart attacks and stroke. This raises the question not only whether Ornish's severe low-fat regimen is the best route for people with heart disease or at risk of it, but also whether it's necessary at all. Even highly motivated people can have a hard time eating less than 20% fat for long—and Ornish's regimen allows for only half of that.

The high-carb content of this diet makes it less than desirable for people with diabetes, who have difficulty controlling their glucose levels. Mounting evidence suggests that people can control their blood glucose on a diet lower in carbohydrate and higher in fat than this plan.

Some of Ornish's claimed evidence is questionable. For example, the thyroid hormone thyroxin, which goes up on Ornish's diet, has actually been found in some studies to slow the metabolism, not speed it up, as he claims. Nor is there conclusive evidence that because dietary fat, compared with carbohydrate or protein, is more easily converted to body fat, low-fat diets—as the author maintains—are more effective for weight loss than other diets. When it comes to weight loss, what counts most is how many calories you take in and how many you burn off. The reason faithful Ornish dieters peel away pounds is simple: They're eating a diet of roughly 1,500 to 1,800 calories a day—low enough for steady weight loss for most people.

Quick fix or lasting results?

This is no quick fix for weight loss; you're in it for life. The goal, Ornish makes clear, should be slow, steady weight loss. Chances are you will experience steady weight loss on this moderately low-cal diet—if you can stick with it. But some degree of fat makes food more palatable, and studies suggest that most people, unless they're highly motivated by the threat of disease, find it tough to sweat out diets as low in fat as this one.

Flexible or rigid?

The Life Choice diet doesn't make you count calories or even fat grams (though fat-tracking charts are included). It pushes no weird food-combining rules, or meticulous schedules, or rules about how many snacks you can or can't have. For a diet to work, Ornish says, it has to be simple and give the dieter freedom to make informed food choices. "The closer you move toward the low-fat vegetarian end of the spectrum," he says, "the greater will be the corresponding benefit." The choice is yours. But the discipline at the end of that spectrum is severe: no meat, chicken, or fish; no added oil of any kind; no sugar; no nuts or seeds; no egg yolks—and only nonfat dairy.

Stumbling blocks

Slashing fat intake to no more than 10% of calories can be a daunting task even for the most dedicated dieter. You'll have to readjust your tastebuds quickly and get used to a whole new way of cooking—preparing onions in stock, for example, rather than sautéing them in oil. Because so few commercially prepared foods have fewer than 2 grams of fat per serving (Ornish's cut-off level for acceptable fat content), you'll be doing a lot of cooking from scratch—a time-consuming task that you'll have to learn to love if you don't already.

Is it for you?

This program may very well be too restrictive for people who relish food in the abundant variety that nature provides. Gourmets, goodbye. Ditto for people with insulin-related disorders such as diabetes. High-carb diets are notorious for sending insulin levels soaring. If you have heart disease, of course, you should be under the care of a physician. It's possible that a diet low in saturated fat, but one that allows a moderate amount of unsaturated fat such as the classic Mediterranean diet, might be healthier for you than Ornish's—and more enjoyable. If you have osteoporosis or risk factors for it, you ought to shop for another diet, or else massage Ornish's program to allow for more dairy products.

Do you have the motivation to overhaul your diet dramatically and write off fat? Then this may be the program for you. It should help you shed pounds, and it may help prevent or reverse heart disease.

Resources

For more on this diet, pick up a copy of *Eat More, Weight Less: Dr. Dean Ornish's Life Choice Program for Losing Weight Safely While Eating Abundantly* (HarperPerennial, 1997), *Dr. Dean Ornish's Program for Reversing Heart Disease: The Only System Scientifically Proven to Reverse Heart Disease without Drugs or Surgery* (Ivy Books, 1996), or *Everyday Cooking with Dr. Dean Ornish: 150 Easy, Low-Fat, High-Flavor Recipes* (HarperCollins, 1997). Additional information is available on Ornish's official website at www.my.webmd.com. Log on if you'd like to participate in live monthly audiocasts with the author.

Fit for Life

Fit for Life is one of the all-time best-selling diet books in the United States. The authors, Harvey and Marilyn Diamond, received their nutrition training at the American College of Health Science, an unaccredited correspondence school in Austin espousing an alternative approach to health known as natural hygiene. According to the Diamonds, it is not what we eat but when and how we eat that matters most in staying healthy and fending off disease. They claim that many thousands of people have lost weight and, more importantly, revitalized their lives by following the principles laid out in Fit for Life and its sequels, Fit for Life II: Living Health and Fit for Life 2000.

The Promise

Basic principles of the Fit for Life plan

If you let waste build up in your body too quickly, the Diamonds believe, you'll develop metabolic imbalances, or toxemia—in their view the source of excessive weight gain and all illness. The underlying goal of the Fit for Life diet is to cleanse the body of such imbalances. You're supposed to eat foods in proper combinations and at specified times during the body's natural 24-hour, or circadian, cycle. If you succeed in following their directives, say the Diamonds, your body will find its natural weight and you'll increase your chance of a long, disease-free life.

The explanation

According to the Diamonds, the body's digestive system goes through three distinct cycles daily. The first, known as appropriation, is the eating and digestion cycle and lasts roughly from noon to 8:00 p.m. Next comes assimilation, when food is absorbed and used by the body. This cycle runs from about 8:00 p.m. to 4:00 a.m.

During the third cycle, elimination, which lasts from 4:00 a.m. to noon, the body rids itself of food debris and body wastes. Under the Fit for Life diet, meals are synchronized with these cycles.

The Fit for Life diet cites three basic eating rules. First, to help cleanse the body you should eat plenty of high-water-content foods (fruits and vegetables). Second, to keep foods from "rotting" in your stomach you shouldn't eat starch and protein at the same meal. (The acids in protein, the Diamonds maintain, cancel out the alkalis in starch, hindering digestion and causing food to sit in the digestive tract, where the food rots and creates toxins.) Third, to whisk fruit quickly through the stomach so that it doesn't produce toxins, you should always eat it on an empty stomach and never with or following another food.

The Fit for Life plan melds the three eating rules with the three daily digestive cycles. Simply stated, the Diamonds recommend that you consume only fruit or fruit juice at breakfast (during the elimination cycle) and that you combine properly foods during midday and evening meals. You're urged to focus on fresh, unprocessed edibles—the less cooked, the healthier—and to eliminate "dead food" from your diet, which includes among other things all animal flesh. "Dead food cannot support life," the Diamonds say. Pasteurization "kills" dairy products, and these and other animal products, they charge, cause high blood cholesterol, arthritis, and osteoporosis as well as contribute to a host of other diseases. So add meat to your list of hands-off items. And while you're at it, avoid foods that have been irradiated, a process that the authors say destroys nutrients.

Evidence claimed

The Fit for Life program is built on the teachings of Herbert Shelton, a naturopathic health practitioner generally considered the founder of the modern "natural hygiene" movement. Shelton promoted the idea of eating only one type of food at each meal and fasting to rid the body of toxins. The Diamonds also cite the writings of John H. Tilden, a physician who used natural hygiene to treat his patients during the first half of the 20th century. Tilden's contribution to natural hygiene: the notion that common cooking methods transform food into an indigestible slag that leaves toxins behind—toxins the body lacks the energy to excrete. Tilden preached that obesity is caused by toxic waste, not by excess calories.

Harvey Diamond jumped onto the natural hygiene bandwagon in 1970 when he applied its methods and disposed of 50 pounds. Since then, he claims, he hasn't had a single headache, stomachache, or cold. Marilyn Diamond, too, says she conquered a variety of health problems and shed 20 pounds by following the principles of natural hygiene.

The Method

How the Fit for Life plan works

The Diamonds outline a two-week Living Health program to launch people on a natural hygiene regimen. The program consists of activities that should be followed six days a week ("dailies") and others that should be followed once a week ("weeklies"). No activities on the seventh, or "breather," day.

One daily is to stick to fruit only in the morning and to combine foods properly during midday and evening meals. You must take special care to separate proteins (meat, dairy products, and nuts) from starches (bread, grains, pasta, and potatoes).

According to the Diamonds, you can continue eating your favorite foods and still lose weight if you eat proteins and starches at separate meals.

You don't have to count calories on this diet. According to the Diamonds, you can continue eating your favorite foods and still lose weight if you eat proteins and starches at separate meals. With each meal you can eat as many vegetables as you like. But remember, you should eat fruit only on an empty stomach and at least 20 to 30 minutes before swallowing other food. In addition, you should drink a glass of water every morning after waking up and another glass five to 10 minutes before each meal. Water, say the Diamonds, will help you control your appetite and wash out any food debris that may be clinging to your stomach lining and digestive tract.

An example of the program's weeklies is "living food" day, when you eat only raw fruits and vegetables, nuts, and seeds ("living foods"). The Diamonds assert that eating raw or very lightly steamed foods for a full day helps the body cleanse itself.

What you'll notice

According to the Diamonds, if you feed yourself correctly your body will do the rest, eliminating toxins and deciding what weight it wants to be. You shouldn't worry if you reach a plateau and stop shedding pounds. The standoff simply means your body is busy doing internal "repair work." Eventually, it will return to the task of losing more weight—if more weight loss is in the stars.

Some people on the Fit for Life diet experience bloating, particularly after eating fruit on an empty stomach. Supposedly, this reaction is fleeting. Eat celery stalks or lettuce with fruit until all toxins have been cleansed from your stomach lining, the Diamonds say, and you'll be able to tolerate fruit on its own.

During your first "living food" day, you may be plagued by hunger, but this usually fades within 24 hours. Afterward you'll feel "lighter, more glowing, and happier," according to the Diamonds. You may also find that you're better able to sleep, focus on mental tasks, and cope with stress.

Additional steps to take

This is much more than a diet. It's a way of life with spiritual overtones. Special breathing exercises, quiet meditation, and sleeping with the window open at night (fresh air helps the body detoxify, say the Diamonds) are some of the recommended dailies in the Living Health program. Weekly activities include long, hot baths, social time with friends, getting to bed by nine o'clock, strolling through the woods, and performing acts of kindness.

The Diet as Lifestyle

Staying the course

The Diamonds present their program as a way of life that will bring "your desires into balance." Sticking with your commitment, they acknowledge, can be difficult. When you first go on the diet you may yearn for your old habits of eating. Take heart. The longer you stay on the diet and follow healthful lifestyle choices, the authors insist, the more steeled you'll become.

Getting into gear

You can't get out of exercise on this plan. The Diamonds recommend a brisk 20-minute walk each day as well as twice-daily stretching sessions and yoga at least once a week. They also tout the benefits of "resistive rebounding," an exercise program that requires a mini-trampoline and one-, two-, or three-pound weights.

Evaluating the Diet

Cautions and concerns

The Diamonds point to success stories as evidence that their approach works. But what happens and why are two entirely different things in this case. It isn't how and when you eat but how much you eat that determines your weight. Strict adherence to the Fit for Life diet will probably lead to weight loss—not because the body is ridding itself of toxins, as the authors insist, but because this is a low-calorie diet and you'll be burning more calories than you take in.

The so-called scientific basis of the Diamonds' approach traces to theories that originated some hundred years ago, when people knew much less about basic physiology and nutrition. The misstatements start with the book's underlying idea—that inappropriately combined foods will "rot" in the digestive tract, causing a buildup of toxic wastes that can make you ill (and fat). No scientific evidence exists to back up this claim. Another false notion is that fruits contain enough calcium to meet your needs even if you've written off dairy. And the idea that digestion uses up more of the body's energy than any physical activity doesn't make much sense.

Some of the advice could be downright risky to your health. For instance, the Diamonds state that the amino acids in egg protein can only be absorbed by the body when eggs are eaten raw, and that unpasteurized milk is more wholesome than pasteurized. Watch out. As food safety experts point out, eating such foods puts you at increased risk of developing campylobacteriosis and salmonellosis, two bacterial illnesses that can cause diarrhea, nausea, vomiting, and headaches. In young children, the elderly, and people with chronic health problems, these conditions can be fatal.

About the only sensible advice in Fit for Life is that you ratchet up your intake of fresh produce. Eating fruits and vegetables to the exclusion of most other foods, however, could be hazardous to your health. The food restrictions here, if followed to the tee, will lead over time to deficiencies in calcium, zinc, iron, and vitamins B12 and D. Moreover, eating fruit only at breakfast could result in poor glucose control.

Quick fix or lasting results?

The Diamonds claim that after an initial adjustment period when you may experience cravings, you'll not only adapt to the Fit for Life program but be transformed by it—"physically, emotionally, spiritually, and psychologically." Don't bet on it. Any diet as low cal as this and with such stringent rules—never eating protein with starch and foregoing all foods except fruit before noon—is likely to defeat the intentions of the most stalwart dieter.

Flexible or rigid?

Though free from counting calories, you'll be wearing a straitjacket of dietary restrictions.

Stumbling blocks

This diet will demand enormous self-control and planning. To help Fit for Life devotees the Diamonds have put together hundreds of recipes, but many contain ingredients that may be difficult to find in your local supermarket. Eating out could also prove difficult; few restaurants offer menu options that meet the program's strict dietary criteria.

Is it for you?

The best weight-control plans are those that teach healthy lifetime habits. You won't find those offered here. Because the Fit for Life diet is deficient in calcium, zinc, iron, and vitamins B12 and D, children, adolescents, and pregnant or breastfeeding women should avoid it. If you're the sort who fades without a full breakfast, hunt for another diet. People with certain types of renal (kidney) disease should also shop elsewhere, as this produce-packed diet may be too high in potassium for them. Are you an overweight but otherwise healthy adult with a great deal of self-control and a loose attachment to meat and dairy products? If so, you might dive into this plan—but consider resurfacing quickly. It should be a temporary regimen only. Make sure you consult your doctor first and take a daily multiple vitamin and mineral supplement, as well as extra calcium.

The Diamonds claim that about half of the people with insulin-dependent diabetes who go on their diet experience "marked improvement" and eventually require less insulin. If this is true, it may have more to do with people losing weight than flushing "toxins" from the body; insulin-related disorders tend to improve with weight loss. No one with diabetes or hypoglycemia should adopt this program with its fruit-only breakfast—which can result in poor glucose control—without first consulting a physician.

Resources

For more on the Diamonds' program, pick up a copy of *Fit for Life II: Living Health* (Warner Books, 1993) or *Harvey Diamond's Fit for Life 2000* (Kensington, 2000) at your bookstore. Marilyn Diamond has also written several recipe books based on the Fit for Life program, including *Recipes for Life* (Avon Books, 1998), *A New Way of Eating from the Fit for Life Kitchen* (Warner Books, 1994), and *The American Vegetarian Cookbook from the Fit for Life Kitchen* (Warner Books, 1990). Information about the natural hygiene movement can be found on the American Natural Hygiene Society's website at www.anhs.org.

The 5-Day Miracle Diet

For more than 20 years Adele Puhn, author of the New York Times bestseller *The 5-Day Miracle Diet,* has avidly promoted the idea that losing weight and keeping it off depends on maintaining stable blood sugar levels. Puhn, a weight-loss consultant, holds a masters of science degree in medical biology and a certificate in clinical nutrition. In her private practice in New York, Puhn claims, she's helped thousands of dieters regulate their blood sugar. Getting off the sugar rollercoaster, she vows, will help you control your weight by jacking up your energy and easing your food cravings.

The Promise

Basic principles of the 5-Day Miracle Diet

According to Puhn, the food we eat, when we eat, and the way we eat all work together to create blood sugar highs and lows throughout the day. Puhn contends that food cravings—those devilish urges that cause you to eat poorly, cheat on diets, or quit them altogether—result largely from depressed sugar levels, a condition she says most of us suffer from. To avoid falling victim to cravings, you have to work with your body chemistry, adjusting it for "good blood sugar" and maintaining it that way indefinitely. By eating specific foods at specific times, and at regular intervals, Puhn promises, you'll eliminate your cravings for starch, sugar, alcohol, caffeine, and fat while increasing your energy, alertness, and sense of well-being. "Give me five days and I'll change your life," pledges Puhn.

The explanation

Puhn's approach is based on some basic facts about how the body processes food to create energy. Blood sugar, or glucose, is the body's main fuel and you have to replenish it regularly. The hormone insulin converts glucose into energy for cell use. Excessive intake of sugar and easily digested starches can spark insulin surges, which in turn can cause blood sugar levels to drop too low as glucose is converted into fat rather than energy. When glucose levels plummet, you feel sluggish and hungry. According to Puhn, your body screams for more sugar to feed and energize its cells. Under such duress, you gobble up anything that sounds appealing, especially carbohydrates like muffins, bagels, pastries, bread, pasta, and candy. These foods are quickly absorbed by your system, giving you a sugar buzz. The effect, however, is only temporary. Soon your body is demanding more calories, usually in the form of sugar and fat. But there's hope, says Puhn. Certain food combinations ensure the proper balance of insulin and another hormone, glucagon, which helps break sugar down into glucose and transport it to the body's cells.

Puhn believes that most of the reason you're tempted to gorge on junk food can be attributed to unstable blood sugar. She also blames a psychological saboteur within yourself whom she calls "Fathead." Emotions such as fear, anxiety, guilt, and low self-esteem can all trigger a diet-busting binge even when you've managed to achieve good blood sugar levels.

Evidence claimed

Puhn's contention that "most of us live in low blood sugar," which creates a mix of physical, emotional, and psychosocial problems, is supported by a 50-item quiz. Five "yes" answers to general questions such as "Do you drink juice as part of your morning routine?" and "Do you experience mood swings?" signal—according to the author—that you're "in bad blood sugar." In her private practice, says Puhn, she has successfully treated thousands of clients with her 5-Day Miracle Diet, many of whom tried and failed on other plans. Her clients come from all walks of life and include CEOs of Fortune 500 companies, actors, socialites, and professional athletes.

The Method

How the 5-Day Miracle Diet works

On Puhn's program you eat breakfast—a serving of protein and a starch—within 45 minutes of waking up. The idea is to begin raising blood sugar levels that dropped during the night while you were fasting. A "hard chew" snack—a crunchy fruit or vegetable such as carrots, celery, or an apple—follows within two hours of breakfast, and a second snack may be necessary if you don't eat lunch within another two hours. Typically, lunch should be eaten no later than one o'clock and should consist of protein and vegetables (a big salad or a stir-fried dish, for example), plus a small serving of a "hard chew" vegetable. By this time you should have achieved balanced blood sugar; the rest of your day is spent maintaining it. Eating one or two more snacks, perhaps a sugary "soft chew" such as grapefruit, at three-hour intervals in the afternoon keeps your blood sugar steady and also keeps cravings at bay during the dicey hours in mid-afternoon when people tend to succumb to the temptation of junk food. A dinner of protein and vegetables should be eaten no later than 8 o'clock if possible. Bread, pasta, and other carbs, which, according to Puhn, can send blood sugar surging, are parceled out sparingly, only on certain days and during certain meals. This schedule balances your glucose levels, she says, and gives the enzymes that break down food a regular routine so they know when to work and when to rest.

The title may mislead you into thinking you'll shed all the weight you want in five days. Wrong. The five days is the time Puhn says it takes to start getting the benefits of good blood sugar. Beyond that, her program isn't divided into specific stages. Abide by her meticulous meal schedule and detailed itinerary of food combos and, you're told, you'll slim down without feeling hungry or lethargic. The personal anecdotes that pepper this book imply that you can expect to lose between one and five pounds a week.

What you'll notice

According to Puhn, it takes 48 to 72 hours for good blood sugar to kick in. She warns that during the first few days your food cravings may be intense. On day one, it is common to feel dizzy and unfocused. On day two, if you're seized by cravings, you're allowed a "hit" of sugar in the form of a small amount of fruit or starch. By day three you'll have more energy and focus, and the food demon will have loosened its hold. You'll also start losing weight. On day four you should be getting into the program's groove, experiencing noticeably less hunger. By the fifth day, Puhn predicts, you'll feel in control of your diet, no longer a slave to the whims of bad blood sugar.

Additional steps to take

The linchpin of Puhn's program is to recognize the feelings that lead you astray. So you're advised to keep a food diary recording when you eat and what, the way you feel, and any outside events that may be affecting how you feel, such as exercise, missed snacks, too much sugar, life's lows and highs. She also advises: Take a multivitamin and mineral supplement with breakfast and a calcium pill at bedtime to make sure you're getting the proper nutrients and to compensate for the dearth of dairy products in her program; drink lots of water, at least eight glasses a day, to remove toxic waste from your body and keep your cells and organs in good shape; weigh yourself only once a week to avoid the emotional rollercoaster of daily weight fluctuation; and limit your salt intake to reduce water retention and prevent high blood pressure.

> The linchpin of Puhn's program is to recognize the feelings that lead you astray.

The Diet as Lifestyle

Staying the course

The 5-Day Miracle Diet is designed to help you not just lose a certain number of pounds but overhaul your eating habits for good. Once your weight goal is achieved, Puhn counsels you to continue abiding by the diet's principles, though you can consume more calories at this point. Exactly how many varies from person to person. Should you be tempted into a sugary, high-fat binge, don't waste your time wallowing in guilt. Instead, Puhn advises, for the next few days make sure you eat your meals and snacks according to schedule and do more exercise. After being on the program for awhile, you'll recover from "relapses" quickly because you'll be so happy with the way you feel when you're in good blood sugar. The knowledge that you have control over your weight will be so empowering, Puhn says; that the feeling of confidence may spill over into other areas of your life.

Getting into gear

Exercise is a crucial part of the 5-Day Miracle Diet. It speeds up your metabolism, relieves stress, helps prevent osteoporosis, burns calories even after you're done, tones muscles, helps you maintain steady weight loss, and elevates your HDL, or "good" cholesterol. Once blood sugar stabilizes, Puhn contends, you'll have so much energy you'll actually want to exercise even if it's not a current practice. If you've been a slouch for ages, she cautions, start slowly. You'll get discouraged if you injure yourself and can't exercise for several weeks. Go walking, pop in an exercise video, pound the treadmill, ride your bike—any exercise that suits your fancy. Begin by exercising one to three times a week, then gradually work up to four or five 30-minute workouts per week. Puhn also stresses the importance of combining aerobic workouts with toning exercises such as weight lifting. For limbering up and relaxing, Puhn offers a custom-designed 15-minute total-body stretch.

Evaluating the Diet

Cautions and concerns

Puhn's approach lays its foundation on generally accepted principles about the action of insulin and how glucose is converted into energy. But then, like those who tout other low-carbohydrate diets (see reviews of the Atkins diet,

The Carbohydrate Addict's Lifespan Program, Protein Power, and *Sugar Busters!*), she makes assumptions that just aren't supported by research. The assertion, for example, that "most of us live in low blood sugar" is misleading. Low blood sugar—in medical parlance, hypoglycemia—is a rare disorder that is not thought to be caused by dietary carbohydrates. Puhn's theory puts the cart before the horse. There is no evidence that excessive carb consumption causes insulin levels to skyrocket and that in turn this leads to obesity. Rather, evidence seems to suggest that obesity can cause insulin imbalances. When you lose weight, these imbalances tend to right themselves, and this seems to be true regardless of how you go about reducing your weight.

Puhn's book is full of before-and-after anecdotes meant to inspire you. If you're looking for harder evidence than that, however, you'll be disappointed. Puhn offers no statistics for the average amount of weight lost by her clients, and no figures for how many of her clients kept the pounds off. And although she hints that her diet is based on careful chemical research into food combinations and their effects on blood sugar, she offers no scientific explanation and doesn't say who the researchers are.

This diet is hardly a miracle. The goal of weight loss should be to improve your health, not make it worse. A three-day sample menu for women measures a meager 825 calories per day, not enough to meet your daily nutritional needs or give you the energy to exercise—no matter what size you are. Puhn discourages consumption of most dairy products because lactose can stimulate insulin production, and bans many high-sugar fruits such as bananas, melons, grapes, pineapples, and mangos, as well as starchy veggies like peas, corn, and acorn squash. She doles out grains sparingly on the grounds that easily digested starches jack up sugar levels too fast. Those who follow this diet to the letter run the risk of osteoporosis from lack of calcium and may be depriving themselves of vitamins and minerals present in forbidden fruits and vegetables.

Quick fix or lasting results?

If you believe Puhn's pledge, on this diet you'll feel better than ever before, and that will motivate you to shed your ugly pounds. "Owning the 5-Day Miracle Diet means this is the way you eat most of the time," says Puhn. So the promised results are supposedly lasting ones, if you stick to the program. But again, the five days are only the beginning: This is not a quick-fix way to lose weight.

Flexible or rigid?

Make sure you have a timer (the eating schedule is micromanaged) and the stomach to handle limited food choices. You will also have to find a way to ensure that you eat 5-Day-Miracle-approved foods at the prescribed intervals. In one sense, however, this diet is flexible: Instead of wasting time weighing food, you can eyeball portions. And Puhn's plan doesn't require calorie counting or shopping for exotic ingredients. Nor do you have to ban certain foods forever. You're allowed "extras" each week—your favorites—but these should be eaten in portions only large enough to satisfy you, and only when you're "in" good blood sugar.

Stumbling blocks

The basic claim that calories don't count is troubling at best. Calories always count when you're trying to lose weight. In defense of Puhn, her recommended serving sizes do limit how much you eat, and there is something to be said for eyeballing portions rather than sweating over calories: It makes eating a less obsessive pursuit. However, if you keep up the food diary for too long, you run the risk of replacing one obsession, calorie counting, with another.

Is it for you?

If you've had your fill of pasta, white bread, and milk and you love to graze, this diet might draw you, if only as a temporary check on fat. But vegetables are the mainstay, so be sure you're willing to take this step. Puhn's assertion that most of us live in bad blood sugar is misleading. If you truly do have insulin problems, you need the advice of a doctor, not this diet.

Resources

Puhn lays out the details of her plan in *The 5-Day Miracle Diet* (Ballantine Books, 1996). She also offers a video to help get you started and an audiotape library with tips on how to manage the regimen on vacation, in restaurants, and at work. To order video or audiotape, or to subscribe to *The 5-Day Miracle Diet Newsletter* and Hotline for the latest news, tips, and menus, call 800-240-6829.

Low-Fat Lies, High-Fat Frauds and the Healthiest Diet in the World

Kevin Vigilante and Mary Flynn are on a mission. Vigilante, clinical associate professor of medicine at Brown University, and Flynn, who maintains a clinical nutrition practice while also teaching at Brown, tout an approach to dieting that avoids extremes and follows some of the most venerable nutritional practices of the developed world. The authors claim that most physicians and most U.S. health agencies, including the American Heart Association and the National Cancer Institute, have become too doctrinaire in their stance against fat. Low-fat diets, the authors argue, are unsavory, unhealthy, and don't work in the long run. But the same holds true, they say, for carbophobic high-fat diets. Vigilante and Flynn's solution: Make Mediterranean cuisine a permanent part of your life, and you'll lose flab and learn to love food at one and the same time.

The Promise

Basic principles

What's wrong with low-fat diets? Not only are they unpalatable and hard to stick to, say the authors, but low-fat diets may impair your ability to absorb vital cancer-fighting nutrients. Moreover, for many dieters low-fat diets can invite heart disease by elevating triglycerides and lowering "good" HDL cholesterol. The trendy high-fat, low-carbohydrate regimens that wishful weight losers have resorted to are equally unsatisfactory. While some people do lose weight on Atkins-type regimens, that's because the dieters are consuming fewer calories, Vigilante and Flynn assert, not because they're reducing or outright eliminating carbs. And watch out for high-fat fraud: All that saturated fat from unlimited beef and butter can clog your arteries.

The answer to the dieter's dilemma is not a weird diet that slashes fat or forbids carbs. It isn't even dieting in the conventional sense. The answer, promise the authors, is learning to respect and relish healthy food—specifically the cuisine of Crete and certain other Mediterranean areas, which is rich in olive oil and plant foods while being light on meat. This type of eating will fill you up on relatively few calories. If you eat Mediterranean and take a brisk daily walk, the authors vow, you'll shave pounds and help stave off myriad medical disorders, among them heart disease, stroke, cancer, diabetes, and hypertension.

The explanation

The seven characteristics of an effective diet, the authors proclaim, are simplicity, palatability and diversity, satiety, nutritional value, durability (has the diet survived for centuries?), universality (is the diet an internationally accepted cuisine?), and harmony (can the diet be easily adapted to your lifestyle and family?). Typically, American weight-loss diets don't fit this bill. "Our diets don't last because we hate them," say the authors.

> The answer to the dieter's dilemma is not a weird diet that slashes fat or forbids carbs. It isn't even dieting in the conventional sense. The answer, promise the authors, is learning to respect and relish healthy food.

But isn't dietary fat the villain that piles on pounds? Why should we eat more of it? Because, Vigilante and Flynn assert, in addition to giving food taste, it makes you feel full longer: Fat slows digestion and stimulates receptors in the small intestine, which signal the brain that you've had enough. "Without a little fat you're always going to be hungry," the authors caution. But you do have to eat the right kind, they point out. The world's healthiest higher-fat diets use added fats like olive oil that can be visually controlled, not hidden fats such as those lurking in doughnuts and bagels.

According to the authors, monounsaturated fat such as olive oil is a nutrition packhorse that contains hundreds of cancer-combating nutrients and antioxidants. In addition to helping prevent the generation of DNA-damaging free radicals, olive oil permits the body to absorb anti-cancer nutrients such as carotenes, which are found in plant foods. If you eat a salad with no-fat dressing, warn the authors, "you're likely to flush most of the cancer-preventing carotenes in that salad right down the toilet." On top of all this, olive oil—as well as other monounsaturated oils such as canola and peanut—helps fight heart disease. It lowers LDL (the "bad" cholesterol that helps build clogging plaque in arteries), and it can maintain or raise HDL (the "good" cholesterol), as well as lowering triglycerides (a form of fatty acid in the bloodstream implicated in heart disease).

Other fats should probably be eaten sparingly, say the authors. Saturated fats, which abound in red meat, whole milk, and butter, don't appear to promote cancer but they do raise levels of LDL. Some polyunsaturated fats—the kind found in corn, soybean, safflower, and sunflower oil as well as most margarines—have been heavily promoted by leading health agencies as a safe alternative to saturated fat. But their tendency to produce DNA-damaging free radicals is reason for caution. The most dangerous fats, say the authors, are trans fats—partially hydrogenated, often-manufactured fats that can dramatically increase the risk of heart disease by lowering HDL and raising LDL. Trans fats are found in French fries, chicken nuggets, and many processed foods labeled low fat, low cholesterol, or healthy.

According to the authors, the inhabitants of the Greek island of Crete consume the healthiest diet in the Western world, with roughly 40% of calories derived from fat, mostly olive oil. That's a hefty 10% above the upper limit recommended by most health experts in the United States. The Cretans also eat an abundance of cereal grains, beans, antioxidant-rich wild greens and fruit, and more limited quantities of goat meat, milk, game, and fish.

Using the Cretan diet as their model, Vigilante and Flynn recommend eating red meat no more than a few times a month because, in addition to being laden with artery-clogging saturated fat, it can contain carcinogens. The authors accuse the USDA of caving in to the meat lobby and encouraging overconsumption of red meat.

In addition to promoting the consumption of more olive oil, less meat, and an abundance of plant foods, the authors recommend drinking a moderate amount of red wine every day—unless you know you're at risk for alcoholism or liver problems. People who drink red wine in moderation live longer and have less heart disease, apparently because red wine, like deeply colored fruits and vegetables, contains phytochemicals that inhibit platelet clotting, cause blood vessels to dilate, and prevent the oxidation of LDL cholesterol.

Evidence claimed

To counter the claims of low-fat-diet advocates, Vigilante and Flynn cite studies suggesting that a low-fat diet is no more effective than any other diet in reducing weight. What expands your waistline is calories, not their source. One study in which European males consumed diets ranging from 25% to 47% fat showed no relationship between percentage of dietary fat and level of obesity.

From this, the authors go on to reason that the moderately high-fat Mediterranean diet, as long as it's low enough in calories, will facilitate weight loss and—because the main source of fat is nutritious, disease-fighting olive oil—promote long-term health.

As evidence the authors cite numerous studies, including the Lyon Heart Study, which showed a dramatic reduction in heart disease symptoms among 300 patients on a Mediterranean diet. In a follow-up study five years later, the same group had a 61% lower risk of cancer and a 56% lower rate of death than a control group. In another significant study of 12,000 men from seven countries—Finland, Greece (including Crete), Italy, Japan, Yugoslavia, the Netherlands, and the United States—men from the isle of Crete were shown to have the lowest rates of heart disease and cancer, as well as the lowest death rates. In northern Italy, where more meat and saturated fat are consumed than in southern Italy, people had higher rates of heart disease. A follow-up analysis revealed that the best predictor of health in the seven-country study was a high intake of monounsaturated fat and a low intake of saturated fat.

The authors also cite abundant evidence suggesting the health benefits of having one to two drinks a day, including the Copenhagen Heart Study of 13,000 people, which showed that drinkers enjoyed a 30% to 40% lower mortality rate than nondrinkers. The authors also review tantalizing, cutting-edge research into the anticancer and heart-healthy effects of red wine.

What about the potential of the higher-fat Mediterranean diet for promoting weight loss? The authors designed a Mediterranean-style weight-loss program and invited 120 people to participate in it. After eight weeks, they claim, all participants reported weight loss ranging from six to 13 pounds, with an average of just over eight pounds total. Many indicated that they dropped pounds without hunger.

The Method

How it works

Vigilante and Flynn offer meal plans and quick, easily prepared recipes for a 1,500-calorie diet for women and a 2,000-calorie diet for men, which can be adjusted up or down depending on individual needs. They also include numerous recipes from restaurants across the country. You won't always have to count calories or puzzle out fat grams. But when you start the diet, the authors advise, you should measure olive oil (a hefty 120 calories per tablespoon), starches, pasta (200 calories per cup), meat, and other high-calorie foods. Eventually you'll be able to gauge reasonable portions by sight. On average, a man trying to shed pounds should consume no more than about 2 tablespoons of olive oil a day, a woman 2 tablespoons. Fruits and nonstarchy veggies can be eaten in almost unlimited amounts. It should be easy to stick to your limits, the authors reassure you, because the sort of Mediterranean cuisine they recommend is filling, in addition to being tasty. If you exercise daily and remain faithful to the diet—better yet, this way of living—you can expect to lose between one and one and a half pounds a week.

> If you exercise daily and remain faithful to the diet—better yet, this way of living—you can expect to lose between one and one and a half pounds a week.

To help you visualize the components of their program, the authors present a Mediterranean Diet Pyramid as an alternative to the USDA Food Guide Pyramid. On the pyramid's bottom two tiers, to be consumed daily, are grains and potatoes, fruits and vegetables, legumes and nuts, olive oil, and cheese and yogurt. Moving up the pyramid, you'll find fish, poultry, eggs, and sweets, to be eaten a few times a week, and on the top red meat, limited to a few servings per month. (See *A Guide to Good Dieting* for specifics on the USDA Food Guide Pyramid.)

What you'll notice

The authors say that in studies of people following their Mediterranean diet, dieters were happy with their food, felt well, and shed pounds at a safe pace. If you have blood tests taken before launching this diet and afterward, you may find that your LDL and triglycerides drop and that your HDL rises—all heart-healthy changes.

Additional steps to take

Vigilante and Flynn aren't demanding: They don't ask you to keep food journals or purchase a warehouse of nutritional supplements. Presumably, you'll be getting all the nutrients you need from the foods they recommend, many of which are fresh, high fiber and plant-based. But the authors do urge you to ban all junk food from your kitchen—including hamburger meat and processed low-fat products—and stock up on Mediterranean ingredients. You need roughly 50 food items on hand at all times if you want to eat healthfully and lose weight on the Mediterranean diet. These include olive oil, cheese, pine nuts, high-fiber bread and breakfast cereal, fresh lemons, canned artichoke hearts, garlic cloves, capers, carrots, green and red peppers, onions, raisins, beans, potatoes, frozen shrimp, lean ham (for occasional use only), canned tuna, canned and fresh tomatoes, and red wine or grape juice. A full list of ingredients is provided so that even the busiest people can equip themselves for just about any Mediterranean-style recipe, even if they haven't shopped recently.

The Diet as Lifestyle

Staying the course

Once you've reached your weight goal, how do you maintain it? Vigilante and Flynn aren't explicit. Supposedly during maintenance you're consuming more calories than during weight loss. It's up to you to determine how many calories will fill you up without filling you out. But the authors do recommend that you train yourself to gauge calories by portion size, a much less taxing approach to dieting than counting calories. This is especially important for dieters who frequent restaurants, where portions—more suited to the appetite of a horse than a human—can quickly sabotage weight control.

How do you keep from bingeing? Go for a brisk walk, advise the authors. Hunger is suppressed both during and for some time after physical activity. "People who ... exercise make better choices when confronted with the temptation to overeat," the authors say.

Getting into gear

We eat too much and exercise too little," Vigilante and Flynn point out, which is why obesity is epidemic in America. While it is difficult to control weight without physical activity, exercise doesn't need to be painful and joyless. Consider the passeggiata—the daily stroll Italians take arm in arm down the streets and through the piazzas of their towns and cities, socializing, shopping, and exchanging news. While it's probably unrealistic to expect fast-paced Americans to adopt this sort of lifestyle, you can make walking a routine part of your life, the authors insist. Start out with 15 minutes of walking every day, they suggest, slowing building up to 30 minutes a day (for improved health and possible weight loss) or better yet, 45 minutes (for almost guaranteed weight loss). If cycling, dancing, gardening, or any other activity holds more appeal for you, fine. In addition to routine exercise, try to make physical activity an integral part of your life by taking stairs instead of elevators or walking to work. "Life," say the authors, "is a journey, and much of it should be traveled on foot."

Evaluating the Diet

Cautions and concerns

The diet that Vigilante and Flynn tout is supported by solid and cogently presented research into the health benefits of olive oil, vegetables and fruits, fish, and red wine. Their comments on the health hazards of low-fat diets, low-carb diets, many processed foods, and polyunsaturated and trans fats also reflect sound science. This diet, diverse and well balanced, should meet most of your nutritional needs while protecting your heart and possibly helping you fight off some forms of cancer.

Can you lose weight on a Mediterranean regime? Yes, as long as you remember that olive oil is a fat and therefore jammed with calories. If you increase your intake of olive oil above the recommended amounts for weight loss, then you'll have to decrease calories elsewhere.

Despite their sensible, science-based approach, Vigilante and Flynn are a little shrill in their attack on the USDA Food Guide Pyramid, charging that it was developed under the influence of the meat lobby and that it hypes meat to the detriment of the public's health. In fact, the pyramid doesn't extol meat to the exclusion of other protein foods. Rather, it suggests that every day you eat two or three servings from any foods in the following group: meat, poultry, fish, beans, eggs, and nuts. What the USDA pyramid fails to do is indicate that daily consumption of red meat, which is laden with saturated fat and carcinogens, may be hazardous to your health.

Quick fix or lasting results?

This approach is a way of life. You'll gradually dissolve pounds while eating a diverse, balanced diet that meets your body's nutritional needs. And if Mediterranean cooking pleases your palate, there won't be any question about sticking with your diet.

Flexible or rigid?

No calorie counting, no food weighing, no diaries, no exotic foods, and no rules that micromanage your day. Just follow the basic guidelines of the Mediterranean food pyramid, watch your portions, and exercise. What could be easier? Even the recipes are user-friendly. Most can be prepared by even a novice cook in under 20 minutes.

Stumbling blocks

Vigilante and Flynn have a loose approach by diet-book standards. Other than advising you to favor certain foods over others, to watch your portions, and to exercise, they're not prescriptive. While this is in keeping with the spirit of their philosophy—the secret to weight control is enjoying food, not obsessing over it—those dieters who prefer being led by the hand through every stage of dieting may feel lost. Others may find that keeping the kitchen stocked with the recommended foods requires frequent trips to the grocery store.

Is it for you?

Farewell fast food and processed junk, hello pasta, pesto, and puttanesca sauce. If can curb your carnivorous instinct, this may be the right approach for you. As with any program, those with special medical problems should consult a physician before starting the Mediterranean diet.

Resources

For more on this style of eating, pick up a copy of *Low-Fat Lies, High-Fat Frauds and the Healthiest Diet in the World* (Lifeline, 1999). If you want personal guidance in following the Mediterranean diet, visit the authors' website at www.meddiet.com.

The Pritikin® Principle: The Calorie Density Solution

Robert Pritikin, director of the Pritikin Longevity Center® founded by his father in 1976, says the key to weight loss is cutting calorie density. Most diet regimens are restrictive, difficult to follow, and unhealthy in the long run, says Pritikin. The Pritikin program is different, claims its author—a simple plan that will help you peel away pounds without hunger and that will also restore or maintain your health. Pritikin says that on his program hundreds of fat-challenged people have achieved a healthy weight and maintained it with ease. Millions more who have read previous books based on the Pritikin Center philosophy, he says, have had the same good results.

The Promise

Basic principles of the Pritikin approach

More than half of the people in the United States are overweight or obese, and the number is increasing every year. Why? Because, says Pritikin, Americans are pigging out on calorie-dense foods and exercising less than in the past. Calorie density refers to the number of calories per weight of food. Peanuts have high calorie density (2,640 calories per pound), tomatoes low calorie density (90 calories per pound). If your diet consists mainly of high-calorie-dense foods such as muffins, dry cereals, granola bars, fried chicken, bacon, and cheese (especially hard cheeses like cheddar), you're destined to put on weight no matter how much you exercise, warns Pritikin, because high-calorie-dense foods tend to have a low satiety value, meaning you have to eat them in large quantity to feel full. But if you add low-calorie-dense foods to your diet, the author goes on, you'll achieve satiety more quickly and reduce total caloric intake. In Pritikin parlance, this is the calorie density solution.

The explanation

According to Pritikin, our urge to stuff ourselves when we're hungry is a primitive, genetically programmed survival mechanism that arose in response to food shortages. It's impossible to overcome this drive, he says, yet that is precisely what many weight-loss programs expect us to do. The trick to weight loss, asserts the author, is achieving satiety on fewer calories. How? By understanding what makes you feel full. As Pritikin explains it, you feel satiated when your stomach contains a certain volume of food, not a particular number of calories. If you know which foods to eat and how to combine them, you can fill your stomach with the same food volume while cutting calories. (Although it is not always the case, there often is an inverse relationship between calorie density and volume: Calorie-dense foods—that is, foods with the most calories per pound—are often the least bulky.)

> The trick to weight loss, asserts the author, is achieving satiety on fewer calories.

Water and fiber add bulk to food, increasing its volume without upping calories. Pritikin claims that consuming foods rich in water and fiber such as fruit, vegetables, and unprocessed whole grains will lower the average calorie density of your meals. In addition to encouraging weight loss, he says, this approach will infuse your body with vitamins, minerals, other nutrients, and fiber. To illustrate the calorie density solution, consider a breakfast of a typical processed cereal like Cheerios. One ounce of relatively low-volume Cheerios has slightly more than 110 calories while an ounce of high-volume strawberries has slightly less than nine calories. Adding the two, you get total calories per ounce: 119. Divide that by two and the average calorie density per ounce is just under 60—much better, Pritikin says, than the 110 calories you started out with. And in all likelihood, you'd probably go for more strawberries than that with your cereal, making the average even better.

Evidence claimed

Pritikin maintains that all the ideas presented here have been tested extensively at the Pritikin Longevity Center in Santa Monica, California. In addition to being a health clinic, this is also a scientific research center devoted to the study of the effects of diet and exercise on health. Pritikin offers motivational stories about clients who arrived at the center overweight, in poor health, and severely discouraged, then rapidly shed pounds and restored their physical and mental health by following the Pritikin program. He maintains that the program battles serious illnesses such as heart disease, hypertension, diabetes, and cancer, and he cites scientific journals in which the results he describes have been published.

Pritikin draws further evidence for the efficacy of his weight management approach from outside studies. The most significant is a 1998 study in which healthy young men were divided into three groups, each of which was fed either a low-, moderate-, or high-calorie-dense diet for 16 days. None of the men knew which diet they were on and all were allowed to eat as much of the food served to them as they wanted. According to Pritikin, the study showed that only the low-calorie-dense group lost weight. The group on the moderate-calorie-dense diet maintained their weight, while the high-calorie-dense diet group gained weight. The study, claims Pritikin, showed that it's more important to be aware of the average calorie density of the meals you eat and keep it below a certain level than it is to count calories.

The Method

How the Pritikin approach works

On this program, you eat three meals a day plus two or three snacks to stave off hunger. Pritikin recommends that you keep the average calorie density of each meal below 400 calories per pound—an achievable goal if you combine foods that are low and high in calorie density and watch your portions. Your diet should consist primarily of whole grain products, veggies, beans, and fruit, with additional foods that are low in fat, cholesterol, and salt. You're allowed three and a half ounces of animal-derived food such as lean chicken or meat and two servings of nonfat dairy each day. (Even low-fat animal products are restricted not so much because of their calorie density, which is moderate, but because of their saturated fat and cholesterol content.)

Pritikin includes a menu guide with suggestions for seven days of breakfasts, lunches, dinners, and snacks. For each meal there are three choices listed—"better," " better still," and "best," rated according to calorie density—along with total ounces, calories, and calorie density. He also provides 52 tried and true recipes from the Pritikin Longevity Center, including salmon mousse, ginger shrimp stir fry, and spiced apple crisp. When planning meals, Pritikin reminds you, the best way to reduce calorie density is to add veggies, since most vegetables contain less than 200 calories per pound. Every carbohydrate such as rice or potato should be served with at least one veggie such as green beans or carrots (Pritikin's "one and one rule"), and every high-protein dish should be served with two vegetables (the "one and two rule"). You can also dilute calorie density with nonfat dairy products.

Pritikin includes a guide for choosing low-calorie-dense restaurant foods as well as a calorie density chart for everything from kidney beans to a variety of processed foods.

121

What you'll notice

By sticking with the program, you're promised, you'll lose weight and have more energy, and your health and quality of life will dramatically improve. Pritikin asserts that many people with serious conditions such as heart disease, adult-onset diabetes, and high blood pressure find that their symptoms disappear after adopting his approach. According to the author, you're likely to sleep better, wake up alert in the morning, look and feel younger, and ease your aching joints.

Additional steps to take

No food diaries or special medical tests are required. Pritikin nutritional supplements can be purchased by calling an 800-number, but they aren't peddled in his book. Beyond dieting and exercise, the author doesn't demand much extra effort.

The Diet as Lifestyle

Staying the course

When you've reached a weight you'd like to maintain, Pritikin advises, you should aim for an average calorie density of between 400 and 600 calories per pound at each meal. This is the break-even point. When you want to cheat—a temptation we're all prone to, admits Pritikin—try "sequencing." Eat your foods in order of their calorie density, working from low to high. You'll be partially full by the time you reach the high-calorie-dense "treats," and thus you'll eat less of them. In fact, it makes sense to sequence at every meal, says Pritikin. If you fall prey to bingeing, you should eat foods almost exclusively low in calorie density for the next few meals. If you really stray far, he counsels, return to the program's recommended menus.

Getting into gear

Humans were designed to move, says Pritikin, and move you must if you want to lose weight and nurture your body. Pritikin recommends walking at least two or three miles a day at a moderate pace of roughly four miles an hour (that is, for 30 or 40 minutes). If the walk can't be completed in one session you can break it up, says Pritikin. Adding weight or resistance training to your regimen will build muscle and help you polish off pounds more efficiently. Don't forget to stretch after exercising, he cautions.

Evaluating the Diet

Cautions and concerns

Pritikin's Calorie Density Solution is the latest twist on the classic low-fat Pritikin program presented in earlier books. This time the approach is essentially a high-carb low-fat diet, heavy on plant-based foods and light on refined carbs, seafood, poultry, and meat. Based on the menus, it appears that Pritikin dieters average 1,500 calories a day with about 10% coming from fat, 65% from carbs, and 25% from protein; standard nutritional guidelines recommend 30% of calories from fat. While low-fat diets have a proven record in reversing heart disease, there are certain risks associated with them. When people go on a low-fat, high-carb diet and they fail to lose weight, their triglycerides (fatty particles in the blood that can damage arteries) go up and their HDL (the "good" cholesterol) goes down—both risk factors for heart disease. Moreover, fat plays a vital function in nutrition delivery: It helps your body absorb cancer-fighting nutrients, minerals such as calcium, as well as vitamins A, D, E, and K. If you radically reduce your fat intake, you could be shortchanging your body of nutrients. Another drawback to low-fat diets is that they can be hard to maintain.

You can address these issues and still stick to the spirit of Pritikin's program. One simple strategy is to augment your percentage of dietary fat (monounsaturated, not saturated) and, by way of compensation, reduce your caloric intake of carbs or protein. The author's advice about consuming plenty of nutrient-packed fruits, vegetables, and whole grains—while watching your intake of refined carbs and saturated-fat-laden foods—is worth heeding if you want to lose weight safely and wisely.

Quick fix or lasting results?

This is supposed to be a steady lifetime commitment, not a high-speed run. If you combine Pritikin's moderately low-calorie program with 40 to 45 minutes of exercise a day, chances are you'll lose weight. Will you keep it off? Yes, if you keep it up. Most people, however, find radically low-fat diets hard to stomach over the long run.

Flexible or rigid?

You'll find this diet fairly flexible—as long as you're willing to slash fat and monitor your meat, poultry, and dairy intake. You don't need to keep track of calories or overly scrutinize portions, though you'll have to become calorie-density literate.

Stumbling blocks

Pritikin's calorie-density chart is extensive but not exhaustive, so you'll be making some calculations of your own. Just one problem: Pritikin doesn't say explicitly how to calculate calorie density. Is your schedule hectic? Then you may find it challenging to consume three low-calorie-dense meals plus two or three snacks every day. And the heavy emphasis on fruit and vegetables might keep you scurrying back and forth to the grocery store for fresh provisions.

Is it for you?

Pritikin's plan calls for only two servings a day of dairy products; those at risk for osteoporosis should either consume more dairy or take calcium supplements. If you're a diehard carnivore, Pritikin's plant-leaning program isn't for you. And if you can't live without pretzels, popcorn, fat-free cookies, and potato chips, you'll struggle with this high-fiber program. People who have elevated triglycerides should eat fewer carbs and more unsaturated fat (olive and canola oil) than the author recommends. Lovers of salad, soup, and whole-grain bread will readily adapt to Pritikin's approach.

Resources

Of nine books that have been written about the Pritikin program since 1979, *The Pritikin Principle: The Calorie Density Solution* (Time-Life Books, 2000) is the latest. For more details on this program or information on the two Pritikin Longevity Centers, log on to www.pritikin.com. You can reach the centers by calling 800-421-9911 (California) or 800-327-4914 (Florida). Pritikin vitamins and supplements can be purchased by calling 800-658-2702; food products can be ordered from the website or by calling 800-238-8090.

Protein Power

Doctors Michael and Mary Dan Eades, authors of the New York Times bestseller *Protein Power*, practice bariatric (weight-loss) and general family medicine in Little Rock, Arkansas. The authors, who have worked with patients suffering from high cholesterol, high blood pressure, diabetes, and obesity, attribute these ailments of modern civilization to a disordered metabolism caused by excess carbohydrates in the diet. They've devised a high-protein low-carb plan that they claim has helped thousands lose weight, lower cholesterol, and get their metabolism running smoothly.

The Promise

Basic principles of Protein Power

Obesity, high blood pressure, elevated cholesterol, and diabetes are all symptoms, say the authors, of an underlying metabolic disorder: excess insulin and insulin resistance. Eating carbohydrates drives your glucose (blood sugar) up, signaling your pancreas to release the hormone insulin, whose primary task is to convert glucose into energy for the cells of your body to use. Insulin helps control your metabolism, telling your body when to burn your food fuel for energy but also when to store it as fat. If your metabolism is working properly, you need just a whiff of insulin to keep your glucose levels normal. However, say the authors, if you rely on carbohydrates as a primary food source, over time you may become insensitive to insulin (insulin resistance), which forces your pancreas to pump out larger and larger amounts of insulin to balance glucose levels. Then, say the authors, this essential hormone becomes a monster. Too much insulin tells the body to store food, not burn it, the authors claim. By eating protein foods and avoiding carbs, you can regulate your blood sugar levels, tame the insulin monster, and control your metabolism.

The explanation

The secret of how the Protein Power approach works, according to the authors, is simple: Get your metabolism to spend more time in the "burn fat for energy" mode rather than the "store fat for later use" mode. The foods you eat, say the Eades, determine which mode you're in. Consuming a high-carbohydrate diet keeps your glucose up and your pancreas pumping insulin, locking your metabolism in the fat storage mode. By contrast, a high-protein low-carb diet prevents your blood sugar from soaring, so your pancreas doesn't have to work overtime cranking out insulin. The result?

Your metabolism spends less time storing fat, say the authors. Protein has this added advantage, they maintain: It signals the pancreas to produce glucagon, a hormone that switches on your burn-fat mode.

By eating protein foods and avoiding carbs, you can tame the insulin monster, the authors claim.

Evidence claimed

The authors contrast the ancient Egyptian diet with the traditional Inuit diet. Examining mummified Egyptian remains, paleopathologists have discovered that the pyramid builders who subsisted on whole grains, fruits and vegetables, fish, fowl, and almost no fat—a diet, ironically, right out of the USDA's Food Guide Pyramid—frequently suffered from obesity, heart attacks, and rotten teeth. Inuit who follow a high protein diet, with little carbohydrate and much fat, experience few heart attacks and have a low incidence of diabetes, obesity, and high blood pressure.

The Eades also cite a study of sorts from 1929-1930 claiming that two Caucasian men who went on a high-protein very-high-fat diet for a year lost about six pounds each and maintained normal cholesterol levels. As additional evidence, the authors cite popular diet books from 1825, 1862, and 1931, each of which promoted a low-carb diet for weight loss, and more recent low-carb diet books by gurus such as Dr. Atkins and the designer of the Scarsdale diet, Dr. Tarnower. Only a diet that worked, reason the Eades, would result in the soaring book sales that these authors have enjoyed.

The Method

How Protein Power works

The Protein Power diet consists of three stages: intervention, transition, and maintenance. Depending on how out of whack your metabolism is, intervention may be broken down into two phases. If you've exceeded your ideal body weight by 20% or more, or have high blood pressure, elevated cholesterol or triglycerides (blood-borne fat), type II diabetes, or glucose intolerance, you start with the phase I intervention. This restricts carbohydrates to 30 grams or less per day (that's equivalent to one bagel) to rein in your rampaging insulin, and usually lasts from four to six weeks. Those with metabolic disturbances such as high blood pressure should wait until their blood pressure, glucose, and triglycerides have been stabilized for at least four weeks before moving on to phase II.

You can skip phase I if you don't have any of the metabolic problems mentioned above or if you plan to reduce your body weight by less than 20%. Phase II intervention allows 55 grams of carbohydrates per day—slightly more than a cup of cooked rice. You're supposed to stay in phase II until you're within 5% of your ideal body weight and your blood pressure, triglycerides, and glucose have remained stable for three to four weeks. Phase I and II intervention is like boot camp, say the authors—strict, grueling, and difficult—but if you stick with it faithfully, you can move on to the next stage and you'll never have to repeat the process.

Do you have to kiss your favorite foods goodbye forever? No, say the Eades.

The next stage is transition, in which you gradually and carefully increase your carbohydrate intake in 10-gram increments until it equals your protein intake or until you stop losing weight. You stay at that carbohydrate level for two months, then slowly increase your carbs in 10-gram increments, waiting five to seven days after each incremental jump to proceed to the next. After each stabilization period you weigh yourself. When you start to gain weight you backpedal to the last level of carbohydrate intake at which your weight remained stable.

At this point you've reached the maintenance stage, where you're supposed to stay for the rest of your life.

What you'll notice

As soon as you switch from a high- to a lower-carb diet, you'll tire more easily and may experience breathlessness. In a few days to a week, the authors reassure you, the fatigue will disappear and you'll start feeling more energetic than before starting the program. Some people experience loose stools and diarrhea a few days into the plan, but usually these problems, say the authors, are resolved quickly. If you were suffering from gastritis, acid reflux (heartburn), or indigestion, they add, you may notice these symptoms disappearing on the diet. Bad breath or a funny taste in your mouth results from the release of ketones in your body, which occurs as fat breaks down. You can alleviate this, say the Eades, by drinking lots of fluids.

Don't fixate on losing pounds in the beginning, advise the Eades: in fact, you may even gain a few pounds if you've been on a low-protein diet for a long time.

As you progress through intervention, your glucose will stabilize, your insulin levels will drop, and you might see a lowering of blood pressure, cholesterol, and triglycerides if these were elevated before. If you have a sweet tooth, your cravings, the authors claim, will ebb.

Don't fixate on losing pounds in the beginning, advise the Eades; in fact, you may even gain a few pounds if you've been on a low-protein diet for a long time. Not to worry—your body's just building muscle that will help you burn fat, they assert. You'll start to lose weight steadily in the intervention stage, about two or three pounds a week. Don't hop on the scale to chart your progress, advise the authors. The scale is misleading because it measures weight, which includes water, fat, and muscle, and what you want to lose is fat, which you can measure more reliably by volume. A better measure of success is to take a piece of clothing that didn't fit you before and try it once a week during the diet.

Additional steps to take

The Eades recommend starting off with a battery of lab tests that will reveal your degree of metabolic disturbance and help you chart your success as your body heals itself through the Protein Power program. These tests should include a chemistry profile to measure blood sugar, potassium, uric acid, cholesterol, triglycerides, and kidney and liver functions. You're also advised to have a serum insulin test, a lipid profile, a hemoglobin test, a 12-lead electrocardiogram, a urinalysis, a complete blood count, and a thyroid panel. You should fast at least eight to ten hours before blood tests.

To avoid the potassium deficiency that might occur on this diet, the Eades advise taking potassium supplements. If you're already taking blood pressure or diuretic medication, check with your doctor before starting potassium supplements. The authors also recommend taking, among other supplements, vitamins C, E, and B complex, beta-carotene, folic acid, iron and calcium.

The Diet as Lifestyle

Staying the course

Once you reach the maintenance stage, you can occasionally stray from the program without suffering long-term weight gain. But only occasionally. To succeed with this regimen you'll have to permanently alter your way of eating. Certain motivational tools can help you, such as eating to stave off ravenous hunger, never skipping breakfast, keeping low-carb snacks handy, and visualizing your goals. If you're tempted to binge on doughnuts, walk away and immerse yourself in an activity, the Eades counsel. Taking action can cause your hunger to evaporate.

Do you have to kiss your favorite foods goodbye forever? No, say the Eades; the key is to decide which meals are the most important in your life—such as Thanksgiving dinner or a birthday feast—then pick a few every year and plan to enjoy them.

Getting into gear

The authors advocate regular exercise, especially lifting weights, to increase the benefits of their nutritional program. Weight training builds muscle, and muscle burns calories to keep you thin. They counsel you to start with light weights, work on the biggest muscles (thighs, shoulders, buttocks, and chest) first, and do the exercise slowly, always on an empty stomach. You can find lots of good books on weight training, but ignore their nutritional advice, warn the authors, because most urge you to load up on carbohydrates. Finally, they caution, don't start exercising until you've been on the plan for at least a week, and remember to crank up your protein intake if you originally calculated it based on a more sedentary lifestyle.

Evaluating the Diet

Cautions and concerns

Like many other diet plans that advocate a reduction in carbohydrates, the Protein Power approach can produce results. The problem—and it's an important one—lies with the reasons given for those results. Indeed, there's little in the way of solid science backing up their conclusions. For example, the authors claim that the type of food you eat determines whether your body burns fat or stores it. However, the overwhelming majority of valid research supports a different conclusion: What determines weight gain or weight loss is how many calories you ingest, no matter what the source—bagels or bacon, butter or bananas—and how many you burn off through exercise. The Eades also maintain that high cholesterol, high blood pressure, and diabetes are caused by carbohydrate consumption. Wrong again. All these conditions are associated with obesity, and all tend to respond favorably to any successful weight-loss program, whether it's high carb, high protein, or somewhere betwixt the two. As for the observation about the high-protein diet of Inuit peoples being healthy because they suffer few of the diseases associated with a carb-based diet, what the Eades fail to point out is that a study done in the late 1970s of the Greenland Inuit showed that they suffer many more strokes than average among the human population. On top of that, there are so many different factors in their lives and their genetic make-up that could play as important a role as diet. The cause-effect relationship just can't be proven with so many variables at work. Furthermore, many of the other so-called studies cited by the authors hardly qualify as valid, especially when they are based on purely anecdotal observation. We've come a long way from two-person study groups from 70 years ago, and even further from diet books dating to the 19th century.

On this diet you're encouraged to eat plenty of nuts, legumes, green vegetables, seafood, cabbage, cauliflower and dairy products—generally recognized as nutritious foods. The downside: You're also given free rein to eat saturated-fat and cholesterol-laden food: egg yolks, butter, beef, even pork rinds for snacking. Fatty foods are the most calorie-dense products you can consume—hardly free fodder for a diet. Worse, saturated fat and dietary cholesterol are linked to increased risk of heart disease. Another downside: For your teensy carb intake you have to choose between the bread/cereal group and the fruit/vegetable group. With the authors rooting for the latter, you're likely to shortchange your body, which needs the energy and nutrients that carbs provide and the disease-fighting, constipation-arresting action of fiber.

Other possible pitfalls: fatigue, nausea, bad breath, dehydration, constipation, and overtaxed kidneys and liver—all common side effects of radically low-carb diets.

Flexible or rigid?

You won't have to count calories and there are few restrictions on fatty foods. But strap on the straitjacket: You'll be poring over carb-content lists and documenting every gram of this supposed poison that passes your lips. If this doesn't put you off the diet, then your body's cravings for carbs just might.

Stumbling blocks

The plan is a bit confusing. In the intervention stage, dieters are told, they should restrict their carb intake to 30 grams a day. Elsewhere they are told that during this stage they'll be cutting out sugar and starches—which, technically, would mean zero grams of carb a day. Moreover, carbohydrates are referred to in grams rather than portion sizes, a difficulty that conversion charts don't go far enough to alleviate. And why, if dieters are allowed unlimited protein, do the authors include protein-equivalency charts? Fooling with charts is one of the diet's drawbacks. As is trooping to the lab for all those tests.

Is it for you?

Vegetarians are welcome: The authors supply alternate protein meals such as tempeh burgers and stir-fried tofu. Those with insulin-related problems might find their blood sugar and insulin levels regulated on this diet. But beware. This diet is radically low carb, and no diet that so severely restricts any of the food groups is healthy over the long term. Don't follow this plan if you're pregnant or have heart disease.

Resources

P*rotein Power* (Bantam Books, 1996) includes an appendix listing phone numbers for purveyors of wild game so you can pack away that protein. And the authors also tell you how to obtain an anatomically correct photo of yourself at your ideal weight to help you visualize your goal. If you want to buy prepackaged protein products, call 800-925-1373 or check out the Eades' website at www.eatprotein.com, which also tells you how to subscribe to the Protein Power newsletter and to enroll as a patient at their clinic. The Eades have written a follow-up book, *The Protein Power Lifeplan*, which expands on their original theory and offers their version of the latest research on insulin.

The Complete Scarsdale Medical Diet

Dr. Herman Tarnower, a cardiologist and founder of the Scarsdale Medical Center in New York, was one of the original champions of the low-carb, high-protein diet. His runaway bestseller, *The Complete Scarsdale Medical Diet*, was first published in 1979. In it Tarnower preached that people could lose up to 20 pounds in 14 days by following his dietary plan. He didn't live long after the publication of his landmark book. He was murdered in March 1980 by Jean Harris, a school headmistress who had been his long-time lover and part-time researcher. Despite the death of its creator, the Scarsdale diet has continued to attract followers, and his book has continued to sell.

The Promise

Basic principles of the Scarsdale diet

In our fast-moving world, says Tarnower, most people want quick results. His program is geared toward pulverizing pounds at an average rate of one per day. Tarnower claims his diet plan can deliver rapid weight loss without hunger because he's unlocked "the mystery of diet chemistry."

The key, he says, lies in eating the right proportions of carbohydrate (34.5%), fat (22.5%), and protein (43%). For comparison, the USDA recommends 60% of calories from carbohydrates and no more than 30% from fat. But according to Tarnower, his mix accelerates the metabolism (the speed at which you process calories, or energy, from food) and turns the body into an efficient "fat-burning machine." Tarnower's regimen is more than high protein and low carb—it's radically low in calories. You should limit the amount of calories you consume to no more than 1,000 a day, counsels the author, at least during the weight-loss phase of the diet. The average recommended by the USDA is around 2,000.

The explanation

If you restrict your carbohydrate and fat intake, Tarnower maintains, your body starts burning fat for fuel. When your body is in this state, known as ketosis, it releases cellular waste products called ketones. According to Tarnower, ketones suppress the appetite. Along with weight, he promises, you'll lose your craving for food.

Evidence claimed

Tarnower says the Scarsdale diet is based on personal "knowledge gained through years of medical practice, day-to-day experience with all kinds of patients, and just plain common sense." He provides no evidence for his claims about the role of ketosis in weight loss, or about the efficacy of a high-protein low-carbohydrate regimen such as his for speeding up the metabolism. Instead, Tarnower settles for enthusiastic testimonials from patients who went on his diet.

The Method

How the Scarsdale diet works

The weight-loss portion of the Scarsdale diet lasts for two weeks. By that point, Tarnower says, your weight should have dipped and your body will need a rest from all its frantic fat burning. Although Tarnower believes most people could remain on his crash diet longer without any ill effects, he recommends against it.

If you restrict your carbohydrate and fat intake, Tarnower maintains, your body starts burning fat for fuel.

On the Scarsdale diet, all your meals are planned for you. You eat the foods the doctor prescribes, and only a few substitutions are allowed. Tarnower does, however, offer several variations on his basic meal plan: "Gourmet," "Money-Saver," "Vegetarian," and "International."

While on the diet your beverages are limited to coffee (black), tea, club soda, diet soda, and water. Alcohol in any form is forbidden. You dress your salads with either lemon or vinegar (no oil) or the vinaigrettes listed in the book. Only lean, skinned, and de-fatted meat are allowed, and veggies must be served without butter or margarine; he recommends lemon juice to add flavor. Between-meal munchies are limited to carrots and celery.

Once you've gotten through your two weeks, you're supposed to stabilize your weight by going on Tarnower's "Keep Trim" maintenance program. This is still a low-carb diet (no potatoes, spaghetti, or rice, for example), but it does permit more foods and calories than the weight-loss program. If you want to continue losing weight, you go back on the crash diet after two weeks of maintenance. Tarnower calls this his Two-On-Two-Off program.

What you'll notice

According to the author, you'll start losing weight almost immediately, to the tune of at least a pound a day. With the hefty drop in weight, he promises, you'll have more energy and an overall feeling of better health. Tarnower also claims that once your body enters ketosis and starts burning fat, your appetite will begin to wane. Despite these gains, he admits, toward the end of your two-week baptism by fire you'll probably be ready for the "food freedom" of the maintenance program.

Additional steps to take

A cornerstone of the Scarsdale diet is the daily weigh-in. Tarnower urges you to keep a written record of your progress during the weight-loss phase. And you should continue monitoring your weight during maintenance, he says. That way you'll know as soon as your weight has increased by four pounds over your desired goal—what Tarnower calls the four-pound stop signal. At that point you'll have to head back to the restrictive diet and stay on it until you've brought your weight down again. Shedding excess pounds shouldn't take more than a week, Tarnower reassures you.

The Diet as Lifestyle

Staying the course

Tarnower claims that his diet, despite its short duration, will help you develop such good eating habits that you'll stay slim for life. His maintenance program offers guidelines for eating in moderation without the fuss of calorie counting or portion weighing. He doesn't say whether you should continue to abide by the same daily percentages of fat, carb, and protein that he recommends for weight loss, but, like the weight-loss portion of the diet, the maintenance stage is still low fat, low carb, and high protein. You're given an extensive list of dietary no-no's, including potatoes, pasta, dairy fat, and all desserts except fruit, and allowed no more than two slices of whole-wheat bread daily. But you can eat cheese, lean meat, shellfish, and salads, and you can have one alcoholic drink a day. His advice for eating out is simply to use good sense: Choose broiled lobster instead of creamy lobster Newburg, for example, and fruit compote instead of a pastry. Tarnower presents a long list of tips for fat-free living, from eating slowly to using nonstick cookware (to decrease your use of fat) and toting around a "before" picture of yourself in a bathing suit.

Getting into gear

A trim, healthy body is the product of a total life style that combines both the right kind of eating and activity," Tarnower says. He advises people to walk at least two miles each day or to find some other nonstrenuous way of expending about 300 calories. Swimming, tennis, and golf are other good options. Tarnower frowns on running because of the increased risk of knee and foot injuries, especially for those over 40. He also recommends against any physical activity that builds huge muscle mass, although he gives no reason for this.

Evaluating the Diet

Cautions and concerns

It's a good thing Tarnower limits his weight-loss phase to two weeks. At 1,000 calories or fewer, it isn't likely to meet your needs for a full spectrum of nutrients. Nor is it likely to set you up for lifetime weight control. This is a crash diet, and most crash dieters are prone to the yo-yo syndrome: After their weight-loss program ends, they put pounds back on with a vengeance. And don't count on Tarnower's promise that you'll lose weight because ketosis suppresses the appetite. Any diet as low as this one is in fat and fiber-rich carbohydrates—proven appetite suppressants—is likely to kindle hunger. A more nutritious, effective way to lose weight and keep it off is to adopt a nutritionally balanced diet, watch your portions, and exercise.

Another concern: Tarnower's program requires that 43% of your daily intake of calories come from protein. This is more than double the amount of protein recommended by most nutritionists. A diet rich in animal protein could elevate your blood levels of homocysteine, an amino acid that has been linked to heart attacks and stroke as well as Alzheimer's disease. Moreover, because your body can't store protein in its dietary form, your liver and kidneys have to work overtime to process it and dispose of the excess. A high-protein diet can cause these organs to enlarge, a risk if you have preexisting liver or kidney disease. Finally, protein tends to leach calcium from your body. People who eat a lot of protein for a long time in excess over a long period of time—and diehard Scarsdale dieters will—may run the risk of developing osteoporosis.

All that protein is consumed at the expense of carbohydrates—another cause for concern. Your body stores carbohydrates with water, and when you slash carbs you can become dehydrated. Indeed, loss of water accounts for some of the rapid weight loss on this diet. Moreover, your brain is fueled by glucose from carbohydrates. In the absence of carbs, the brain gets its glucose from muscle protein. Thus some of the weight you shed on this diet could be muscle. Loss of muscle mass can result in fatigue and a disinclination to exercise. Since exercise is one of the cornerstones of lifetime weight control, you should seriously question any diet that limits your ability to be active.

Other conditions that can be caused or aggravated by high-protein low-carb diets such as this: gout, gallbladder stones, constipation, bad breath, nausea, and dizziness.

Quick fix or lasting results?

This can be the fast track to weight loss. But if you zap pounds, it's not because of any special ratio of fat to protein to carb—as Tarnower claims—but simply because your calorie intake has plunged. Almost anyone who takes in only 1,000 calories or fewer a day will lose weight quickly. Experience shows, however, that rapid weight loss often results in rapid weight gain. Tarnower's vow that his diet will preserve your svelte figure year after year is questionable.

Flexible or rigid?

For the first two weeks you'll be glued to Tarnower's menu plan—remember, no substitutes. Thereafter you'll have to avoid foods on a long list of no-no's. Still, you won't have to count calories or weigh foods, and once you're in the maintenance stage the list of allowable foods will give you some flexibility in meal planning.

Stumbling blocks.

During the two-week weight-loss phase, you'll be following a tight, time-consuming blueprint as you plan meals, shop, and cook—especially if you're the chef in the family and protesting members demand separate meals. Numerous food restrictions could make this diet difficult to follow when you eat out or travel.

Is it for you?

If you're looking for rapid weight loss, you don't have any medical problems other than excess pounds, and you can survive temporarily without sugar, chocolate, pasta, potatoes, and any number of other mouth-watering foods, you might try this program as a temporary assault on fat. But be sure to consult your doctor first. And after those two weeks, you'd probably be better off going on a more balanced maintenance diet—more complex carbs, less protein—than the one Tarnower recommends. If you have gout, kidney or liver disease, gallstones, diabetes or risk factors for osteoporosis, or if you're pregnant, you should avoid this diet and see a doctor before going on any other.

Resources

You can learn more about the Scarsdale diet by picking up a copy of *The Complete Scarsdale Medical Diet Plus Dr. Tarnower's Lifetime Keep-Slim Program* (Bantam Books, 1995).

The Schwarzbein Principle

Dr. Diana Schwarzbein is an endocrinologist whose work with type II diabetes convinced her that a low-fat, high-carbohydrate diet leads to poor health and excess weight. Schwarzbein has her own controversial take on the reduced-carb diet touted by many diet gurus. Following the Schwarzbein diet, people eat protein and "good" fat to their stomach's content—à la the Atkins approach—but cut out all processed and refined foods, salt, caffeine, alcohol, and artificial sweeteners as well as sugar. Founder of the Endocrinology Institute of Santa Barbara, Schwarzbein claims to have helped more than 3,000 patients improve their health and lose weight by putting them on her nutrition and lifestyle regimen.

The Promise

Basic principles

According to Schwarzbein, high insulin levels caused primarily by eating too many carbs (resident in sugar, grains, fruits, some vegetables, and most dairy products) are the main reason so many Americans are overweight. Schwarzbein links insulin to many of the degenerative diseases associated with aging, such as osteoarthritis, diabetes, heart disease, and certain cancers. The underlying goal of the Schwarzbein program is to tame insulin levels through carbohydrate cutbacks and other lifestyle changes.

The connection Schwarzbein makes between carbohydrates and insulin traces to some basic facts about metabolism. When you eat carbohydrates your blood sugar, or glucose, rises. Insulin is the hormone that regulates the conversion of glucose into energy for use by your body's cells. Schwarzbein maintains that if your insulin levels stay too high for too long you become insulin resistant: The hormone no longer performs its main function properly and instead converts more and more glucose into fat. In addition, hormonal imbalances, says Schwarzbein, lead to widespread cell damage or "accelerate metabolic aging." Metabolic aging happens to each of us as we grow older, Schwarzbein asserts, but prolonged high insulin levels can accelerate the process. For this reason, she says, "people are getting fatter, sicker, and more depressed."

How to tame runaway insulin levels? According to Schwarzbein, put a check on your carb consumption and indulge in as much protein and "good" fat as you like. Schwarzbein's blanket okay to eat dietary fat—including saturated fat—is based on the notion that calories from dietary fat as opposed to other sources are less likely to morph into body fat. Her platter is crowded with butter, mayonnaise, eggs, and other foods that used to be hands off for dieters. But her program is not a passport to complete abandon. Not only do you wean yourself from carbs, which means no foods made from refined flour, but you also cut out caffeine, salt, alcohol, sugar, artificial sweeteners, and processed edibles of every sort. You should confine yourself to unprocessed, or "real," food—that which in theory can be picked, gathered, hunted, or fished.

The explanation

Schwarzbein argues that insulin resistance—a recognized medical condition—is acquired, not inherited and therefore can be reversed. In this she differs with other advocates of low-carb diets, such as the authors of *The Carbohydrate Addict's Lifespan Program*, who blame a genetic predisposition for insulin resistance; it should be noted, however, that even those who claim the problem is inherited say it can be corrected through diet. For her part, Schwarzbein explains that her nutritional program works by lowering insulin levels, which eventually reverses insulin resistance and heals the body's metabolism. The idea is that once your metabolism begins to heal, your cells start using up your body's stored fat, and you lose weight.

Evidence claimed

Schwarzbein relies heavily on clinical experience. She began developing her theories while working with people who suffer type II diabetes, also known as adult-onset diabetes, a condition that typically involves insulin resistance. When she switched these patients from standard low-fat, high-carb diabetic fare to her low-carb, high-fat program, Schwarzbein claims, they underwent dramatic changes in their health, achieving normal blood sugar levels, lowering their cholesterol levels and blood pressure, reducing body fat, and building muscle mass. Buoyed by this success, Schwarzbein began testing her program on nondiabetic patients, who, she says, were soon reaping similar benefits.

According to Schwarzbein, there are no long-term studies showing that low-fat diets are actually good for you. But, she says, there is plenty of research linking high insulin levels to heart disease, high blood pressure, and obesity—proof, she claims, that low-carb diets are healthy. Schwarzbein believes high insulin levels—and the diseases they trigger—are a direct result of poor eating and other lifestyle habits. Because poor habits are becoming more widespread among the young, in her estimation, conditions once associated only with aging such as type II diabetes and obesity are now showing up in younger and younger people.

The Method

How the Schwarzbein Principle works

Schwarzbein prescribes two different nutritional programs, one for "healing" and one for maintenance. Trimming down is most likely to occur during the healing program as you hold carbohydrates in check. Schwarzbein offers several guidelines for this phase: Never skip meals; stick to unprocessed food (those that can be picked, gathered, hunted, or fished); include fats, proteins, nonstarchy vegetables such as leafy greens, and a limited amount of carbohydrates in each meal; and avoid caffeine, alcohol, and drugs, including over-the-counter and prescription medications. Of course, always be sure to check with your physician first before stopping any prescribed medication.

On the Schwarzbein plan, you don't have to weigh foods or count calories or fat grams. Focusing on numbers can create an obsession with food, says the author. She does offer guidelines for how many carbohydrates you should eat during healing, however. Those numbers are determined by your weight and your activity level. A slightly overweight person who is somewhat active, for example, should take in 15 to 30 carbohydrate grams per meal—an amount that is equivalent to no more than one plain bagel or less than a cup of rice.

How long you stay on the healing program is up to you, although Schwarzbein is quick to add that you shouldn't follow it for life. If you're more than just slightly overweight, she says, you can expect to cast off one to two pounds a week while healing. Some people's metabolisms, however, are so ravaged that burning fat takes much longer. In that case, she predicts, you won't lose weight for six months to a year, and you may actually gain weight at first.

Once "your symptoms are alleviated or your illness is healed," you should move on to the maintenance program, similar to the healing phase except that now you can gradually ratchet up the carbs.

What you'll notice

You may feel hungrier after launching yourself on this program, but according to Schwarzbein that's a good sign: It indicates that your metabolism is improving. You may also experience indigestion, bloating, gas, constipation, and water retention. Eventually your body will adjust to the new eating regimen, says Schwarzbein, and you'll notice a host of benefits: improved sleep, more energy, better concentration and memory, fewer food cravings, and an increased libido. If you're one of the people whose weight stays constant or goes up slightly, your body will still look and feel better, she vows. Your mood will also improve because you'll be feeding your brain a steadier supply of serotonin, the brain chemical that induces a sense of well being. In addition, Schwarzbein claims, your immune system will strengthen, translating into fewer bouts with colds, flu, and other illnesses.

Additional steps to take

Although Schwarzbein believes the best way to get vitamins and minerals is from real food, she acknowledges that some people need supplements—and she recommends a pharmacy-sized list. Some of her suggestions: a multivitamin and 1,000 milligrams of calcium once a day; 1,000 milligrams of essential fatty acids twice a day; a stress-reducing B-complex vitamin and 250 to 300 milligrams of St. John's wort each morning; in the evening, 250 to 500 milligrams of magnesium; either 250 to 500 milligrams of L-tryptopha (prescription only) or 25 to 50 milligrams of 5-hydroxytryptophan (5-HTP) (over the counter); and finally, to help your body adjust to the new foods you're feeding it, digestive enzymes such as papaya tablets.

Because aging can wreak havoc on the body's hormones, some people may need hormone replacement therapy, says Schwarzbein. She advises seeking out a physician who uses "real" hormones—identical to those found in the human body—rather than synthetic ones. Real hormones include estradiol, progesterone, testosterone, and levothyroxine (thyroid hormone). To get insulin and other hormone levels balanced, stress management is helpful, Schwarzbein contends. She recommends a variety of methods for lowering stress, from aromatherapy to meditation and prayer.

The Diet as Lifestyle

Staying the course

The maintenance program is similar to Schwarzbein's healing program, except you don't have to keep your carb intake below your metabolic needs. What are those needs? That's up to you to determine. Supposedly you can tell when your metabolism is off-kilter by symptoms such as fatigue and a host of ailments that includes acne, allergies, headaches, and chronic yeast infections. Once you're on the maintenance program, says the author, if any of these conditions reappear you should decrease your carbs again and hustle yourself back into healing.

Getting into gear

Exercise is "vital," says Schwarzbein, and you should fold it into your daily routine. Start slowly if you're out of shape, perhaps by walking for five minutes three times a day. Gradually extend your workout to 15 to 20 minutes three times a day, or exercise for a single longer period. The best time to exercise, she says, is one to two hours after eating. Schwarzbein suggests moving at a pace that raises your pulse to 60% to 80% of your maximum attainable heart rate (to arrive at this figure, subtract your age from 220).

If you're exercising regularly you're allowed to increase the amount of carbohydrate in your diet. But Schwarzbein warns against carb-loading for optimum performance—a practice popular among athletes—claiming that carb-loaders are no match for athletes who eat a more balanced diet.

Evaluating the Diet

Cautions and concerns

The Schwarzbein Principle is yet another version of the wildly popular low-carb diet, and like the others it can indeed produce results. The fault, however, lies in the reasoning—a flaw that calls into question the diet's entire approach. Schwarzbein argues that a high-carb diet leads to high insulin levels, which in turn leads to excess padding (particularly around the waist). Therefore, the logic quite naturally seems to be, reduce carbs. This theory, though compelling, has no scientific basis. Calories are what pack pounds, not carbs or insulin. Are calories from dietary fat less likely to convert into body fat than calories from other sources, as Schwarzbein would have you believe? No. And her notion that being insulin resistant raises your chances of becoming overweight is misguided. Reverse the order: The chubbier you are, the greater your risk of developing insulin resistance (and type 2 diabetes). Lose weight and your insulin problems may self-correct.

Dieters should beware of Schwarzbein's free ticket to dietary-fat heaven. Other than genes, the major determinant of LDL—the villain cholesterol that clogs your arteries—is the amount of saturated fat in your diet. Diets brimming with foods like butter, eggs, and mayonnaise (all on Schwarzbein's "good" fat list) have been clearly linked to heart disease, not to mention obesity and certain cancers. Most nutrition experts recommend restricting saturated fat intake to 10% of your calories. On Schwarzbein's diet it's easy to exceed that limit.

The lurking land mines of a low-carb diet are many. Cutting back on carbs—your body's preferred fuel source—may lead to fatigue and hamper your ability to exercise. During World War II Canadian infantry troops were given tea and pemmican, a type of beef, as emergency rations; virtually deprived of carbs, the men grew listless after three days and didn't recuperate until carbs were reintroduced into their diet. Low-carb regimens can also slow down your plumbing. Most Americans already eat much less fiber than the 20 to 35 grams that most nutritionists recommend, and on this diet no doubt you'll be ingesting even less. Perhaps most seriously of all, you can put your kidneys and liver at risk on a diet that is high in protein: These organs could enlarge as they put in overtime processing large amounts of protein. Other possible pitfalls associated with low-carb diets: nausea, headache, bad breath, and calcium loss, which can lead to osteoporosis.

Quick fix or lasting results?

Depending on your body type, you could lose weight within a few short weeks or you could tap your fingers for months before noticing any change. Regardless of how long it takes, the author would like you to stick with her maintenance phase for life. Is that possible? Diets that limit food groups inevitably lead to cravings for banned foods. You may well lose weight on this diet, first by water loss and then through decreased caloric intake owing to the monotony of the food choices, but remember, monotonous diets tend to self-destruct. Humans have an appetite for a variety of victuals, a characteristic that encourages consumption of the full spectrum of nutrients. Can you slash back your intake of pasta, bread, and other carb-rich foods and stand it for a lifetime? Unlikely.

Flexible or rigid?

This diet is flexible in in that it authorizes unlimited amounts of protein and "good" fat. But sorry, no fatty fast foods—in fact, no processed or refined foods of any kind. The long list of other no-no's, such as caffeine, salt, sugar, and artificial sweeteners, may make the diet too rigid for some wishful weight losers. The sunny side: You needn't worry about counting calories, only carb grams—and then only during the healing part of the program. In fact, Schwarzbein admonishes her dieters not to become obsessed with numbers, not even those on the bathroom scale.

Stumbling blocks

You'll have to count carbs, at least during the healing phase. If you've got the temperament for details, fine. You could lose your way during the maintenance phase, however, because Schwarzbein doesn't say how many carbs you should ultimately be ingesting in order to maintain a healthy metabolism. Determining the proper level might entail a lot of frustrating trial and error.

Do you like to cook, and do you have time to spare? Good, because you'll be working with whole foods instead of zapping processed food in the microwave. If you're cooking for others and can't convince them to swallow the same spartan low-carb diet that you've adopted, this regimen could prove to be an intricate juggling act.

Is it for you?

If you've got a sweet tooth, steer clear—there's no assuaging it on this ban-all-sweeteners diet. Those with insulin-related disorders should check with the doctor before attempting this approach. Many insulin-resistant people can control their problem by going on a much less restrictive diet than this, one that only limits carbs to 45% of the diet; if you're consuming 2,000 calories a day, that would translate to 225 grams of carb.

Schwarzbein's program is not for pregnant women or people with gout, kidney, or liver disease, osteoporosis, heart disease, or risk factors for these conditions such as family history. Meat eaters, of course, are welcome. So are vegetarians, although not those who restrict all animal products: They can substitute eggs, cottage cheese, peanut butter, and tofu for meat.

Resources

· ·

For more on Schwarzbein's nutritional program, pick up a copy of *The Schwarzbein Principle*, co-authored by Schwarzbein and Nancy Deville (Health Communications, 1999), *The Schwarzbein Principle Cookbook* (Health Communications, 1999), or *The Schwarzbein Principle Vegetarian Cookbook* (Health Communications, 1999) at your local bookstore.

Suzanne Somers' Get Skinny on Fabulous Food

Suzanne Somers, author of *Get Skinny on Fabulous Food* and other bestselling diet books, is also a television actress and founder of the Suzanne Somers Institute for the Effects of Addiction on Families. Her "Somersizing" plan targets what many popular diets say is the real enemy of weight loss: not fats, not proteins, but carbohydrates. Somers claims that more than one million people have slimmed down marching to the tune of her high-protein, high-fat, low-carb diet.

The Promise

Basic principles of the Somers approach

According to Somers, eating fat doesn't make you fat—or diseased. Her mantra: "Fat is your friend." If you cut too much fat out of your diet, she says, you'll slow down the production of necessary hormones, accelerating "metabolic aging" and increasing your risk of illness. The foods you should be wary of are certain carbohydrates. Sugars and high-starch foods such as white flour, white rice, and potatoes, says Somers, are a dieter's worst nightmare because they cause hormonal imbalances that lead to weight gain.

In addition to avoiding carbohydrate villains, you should eat foods in proper combination, Somers cautions. Proteins and fats should be consumed separately from carbohydrates, and you should avoid eating fruit with other foods because it causes gas and interferes with digestion. Somersizing involves no calorie counting or portion control. You can eat until you're full—so long as you eat the right foods in the right combinations.

The explanation

Somers is a devotee of the dietary theory espoused by Diana Schwarzbein, M.D. (see the review of *The Schwarzbein Principle*). That theory founds itself on some basic information about how the body metabolizes food. When we eat carbohydrates, they are broken down into glucose, or blood sugar—the body's preferred fuel. As glucose levels rise, so do levels of the hormone insulin, which is produced by the pancreas. Insulin is responsible for converting glucose into energy for the use of our body's cells. According to the theory Somers touts, carbohydrates can cause insulin levels to get too high, in which case the body no longer responds to the hormone properly—a recognized condition known as insulin resistance—and insulin levels increase even more. In this state, instead of being converted into energy, excess glucose becomes stored as body fat. To control the problem, goes the theory, you need to get insulin levels to normal, and you do this by reducing your intake of foods that raise glucose levels. Somers classifies foods according to their glycemic index, or how fast they break down into glucose. You should steer clear of edibles that fall at or near the top of the index such as sugary foods and many starches—in other words, most carbohydrates. Those that fall near the bottom—natural fats and proteins—can be consumed with abandon.

> Somers vows that her diet will cause your digestive system to operate "like clockwork."

Somers vows that her diet will cause your digestive system to operate "like clockwork." By eating the right foods in the right combinations, you'll enable your body to get the nutrients it needs and quickly discard the rest. As a result, she says, you'll lose weight and have more energy.

Evidence claimed

The Somersizing diet is based almost exclusively on the Schwarbein Principle. Schwarzbein, a California endocrinologist who has worked with patients suffering from type II, or adult-onset, diabetes, wrote the foreword to *Get Skinny on Fabulous Food*. She claims that the low-fat, high-carbohydrate weight-loss diet accepted by most members of the medical establishment has no scientific foundation. There is scientific evidence, she counters, proving that high insulin levels are linked to heart disease, high blood pressure, obesity, and other health problems. Her conclusion: The best way to keep insulin levels and weight down is to cut back on carbs.

Somers backs up her diet plan with impassioned testimonials, trotting out personal letters and before-and-after photos from many of her readers. She herself dropped 14 pounds on a Somersizing diet, while her husband, following the same regimen, brought his cholesterol from 265 down to 178 and chucked his cholesterol-lowering medication.

The Method

How the Somers approach works

The Somersizing diet has two levels, weight loss and maintenance. During level one, you eliminate "funky foods" that cause blood sugar levels to get out of whack. Funky foods include sugar, refined (white) flour and rice, starchy fruits and veggies such as carrots, potatoes, bananas, and acorn squash, as well as caffeine and alcohol. You should also scratch from your list all "bad combo" foods—those that pack protein with carbs, or fat with carbs. Among those foods to be avoided at all cost are nuts, olives, avocados, tofu (unless you're vegetarian), milk, and yogurt.

Somers divides acceptable foods into four groups: "pro/fats," or foods that combine protein and fat, such as meat, poultry, fish, eggs, as well as "natural" fats such as oil, butter, cream, and cheese; fresh vegetables, but only those that are low in starch, such as leafy greens; fresh fruit, but no bananas, which have a significant amount of carbohydrate; and a relatively short list of acceptable "carbos," including whole-grain breads and pastas, beans, and nonfat dairy products. Fruit must always be eaten alone, on an empty stomach. Pro/fats can be eaten with veggies, as can carbos, but pro/fats and carbos shouldn't be consumed together. You're supposed to wait three hours between a pro/fat and a carbo meal, eat at least three meals a day, and never skip breakfast. Portions are up to you, although Somers recommends eating only until you feel "comfortably full."

Once you've reached your goal weight and "healed your metabolism," you're ready for level two, lifetime maintenance. Now you can return to eating funky foods and combining pro/fats and carbos, but only occasionally and in moderation. The freedom to eat unlimited amounts is now curbed; during level two you limit portions to keep from regaining.

What you'll notice

You may crave carbs during the first few days of the Somersizing diet. This will diminish, Somers promises, "as your system unloads the built-up sugar from your cells," and soon you'll be energized and losing weight. Some Somersizing dieters manage to cast off five or more pounds the first week, she claims; others don't see any results for up to one month. Somers promises that no matter how much you eat, you won't feel stuffed or bloated on her diet because you'll no longer be bombing your digestive tract with bad food combos. However, bloating, carb cravings, energy dips, and extra pounds may return during level two when you reintroduce eating practices banned during level one.

Additional steps to take

Somers recommends buying fresh and whole grain rather than processed or refined foods. Processed foods, she says, contain free radicals, molecules scientists have recently implicated as key players in the aging process. Somers also recommends drinking eight to ten glasses of water each day, preferably between meals, rather than during meals or right before you eat.

The Diet as Lifestyle

Staying the course

Finding your dietary "equilibrium" is what level two, or the maintenance stage, is all about. During maintenance you can reintroduce specific foods or food combinations, but only so long as your body tolerates the change. As soon as you notice your energy sagging, your body bloating, or the pounds piling back on, you should backtrack to level one. Beware of slipups, Somers cautions: One sugar-laden dessert can soon lead to another, until "before you know it, you've started adding bad combinations and a little white flour here and there." To stave off a sugar craving, she suggests nibbling on a pro/fat food such as cheese to help stabilize blood sugar levels.

Getting into gear

Somers advocates regular exercise without getting into specifics. Her motto: "Be fit, not fanatic." On hectic days when a structured workout isn't possible, she says, you should build physical activity into your routine. She suggests things like playing tag with your kids or taking stairs instead of the elevator. Somers describes part of her own exercise regime: three 30-minute weight-resistance sessions a week under the tutelage of a personal trainer.

Evaluating the Diet

Cautions and concerns

Diets such as Somers' that severely limit carbohydrates can cause you to lose weight. The important issue, though, is why, and that's where the advocates of low-carb dieting tend to go astray. High insulin levels do increase the risk of heart disease, but despite the claims of Somers and others, there is no scientific evidence that high insulin levels from eating carbohydrates cause people to store fat. For most people who do not have an insulin disorder, the insulin response to carbohydrates—even a dramatic rise—is short-lived and the body accommodates it like a finely tuned machine. Carbohydrates are no more likely to contribute to weight gain than any other food that you eat to excess. When it comes to dieting, the refrain is familiar but nonetheless valid: It's calories that count—whether they come from carbs, fats, or proteins.

As for the theory about food combining—an offshoot of a movement that originated a century ago when people knew little about physiology and nutrition: No evidence exists of any benefit to be derived from eating fruit alone or consuming proteins and fats separately from carbs.

The biggest potential danger here is Somers' argument that the more "good" fats you eat (in the form of butter, oil, cheese, sour cream, meat, and fish), the healthier you'll be. It borders on irresponsibility to trumpet this message in light of the number of studies that have linked a high-fat diet to obesity and cardiovascular diseases such stroke atherosclerosis. This is a low-carb diet high in fat and protein, and dieters should beware of the possible health risks associated with such an imbalance. Among other conditions, too little carbohydrate can lead to dehydration, constipation, fatigue, gout, and nausea. Too much protein can result in kidney or liver damage and, possibly, calcium loss.

Somers is a better guide when admonishing her readers to cut back on refined sugar, which is high in calories and low in nutrients. Americans eat far too much sugar, often hidden in processed junk food. If you ferret out and eliminate excess sugar from your diet, your waistline may well thank you. But you'll have to rein in the calories from fat and protein as well.

Quick fix or lasting results?

Alifestyle that allows you to enjoy food, rather than fear it" is how Somers defines her diet plan. Indeed, Somersizing gives you permanent license to graze on protein and calorie-dense fat. Butter, steak, eggs, cheese—sound like heaven? Maybe so, if you can develop a take-it-or-leave-it (mostly leave-it) attitude toward carbohydrates. The question is, over the long run is it healthy to eat as much saturated fat as this diet encourages, and when you tire of all the fat and protein, will you high-tail it back to carbs?

Flexible or rigid?

No counting calories or sweating over portions on this diet—at least during the weight-loss stage. But the slash-and-burn approach to carbs, the wrenching of proteins and fats from carbs, and the rule about consuming fruits all by their lonesome? These restrictions may prove too much in the long run for even the most diehard dieter.

Stumbling blocks

You'll have to rigorously limit your carbs, be vigilant about food combining, and avoid Somers' "funky food" hit list. All this makes the old-fashioned business of calorie counting sound easy by comparison. Busy people or those who are living in a household with others not as enamored of this diet may find its rules challenging.

Is it for you?

Your antennae should go up whenever an uncredentialed diet crusader says to avoid milk, yogurt, bananas, carrots, avocados, and acorn squash—all of which have nutritional benefits—and to go for the butter, red meat, cream, and cheese. If you exercise frequently, cutting back on carbs, the body's fuel of choice, will zap your energy. The high intake of saturated fat on this diet may turn you into a ticking time bomb for heart disease. As for those with risk factors for osteoporosis: Don't even consider this diet. Milk and yogurt are taboo, and because the regimen is high in protein it could leach calcium from your system. Think twice before Somerizing if you've got gout or kidney or liver disease. With all these provisos, for most people it would be far safer—and simpler—to eat a balanced diet in moderation and exercise your excess calories away.

Resources

For more on Somersizing, pick up a copy of *Get Skinny on Fabulous Food* (Crown Publishers, 1999) or *Eat Great, Lose Weight* (Three Rivers Press, 1999). Somers is the spokesperson for a line of fitness products. You can order the basic product and a training video on the Web at infomercialindex.net.

Sugar Busters!™

Three Louisiana doctors and a CEO teamed up to write this *New York Times* bestseller, which blames obesity on sugar consumption. Businessman H. Leighton Steward, heart surgeon Morrison Bethea, endocrinologist Samuel Andrews, and gastroenterologist Luis Balart urge readers to slash their sugar intake to shed pounds and achieve healthy cholesterol levels. The authors claim you can lop off weight and keep it off simply by eliminating certain carbohydrates—the food group to which sugars belong—from your diet. The Sugar Busters!™ icon: a sugar cube with a red slash through it.

The Promise

Basic principles of Sugar Busters!

By cutting out sugar, the authors claim, you can consume more calories than before and still lose weight. What's being busted here isn't just table sugar, however. Brown sugar, corn syrup, molasses, and honey are also no-nos. White flour, white rice, and most pastas don't pass muster either. Nor do such seemingly nutritious foods as potatoes, corn, carrots, and beets. Why are these foods taboo? Because they are quickly broken down in your digestive tract to glucose, the basic form of sugar that your body uses for producing energy.

The explanation

Sugar causes your pancreas to produce the powerful hormone insulin, which regulates glucose levels in your bloodstream and is responsible for converting blood sugar into energy. When you consume too much sugar, say the authors, your pancreas pumps too much insulin, which stores excess glucose as fat. Not only does insulin store fat, they add, but it also prevents the body from breaking down

No matter how carefully you count calories or how often you exercise, the reasoning goes, a high-sugar diet will keep you from losing weight.

previously stored fat. So no matter how carefully you count calories or how often you exercise, the reasoning goes, a high-sugar diet will keep you from losing weight.

Instead of products like white bread, cookies, and pizza crust, the authors recommend that you increase your consumption of whole-grain foods. They're an acceptable type of carbohydrate because they are digested more slowly, and thus keep insulin levels lower overall. Other high-fiber foods such as dried beans, green vegetables, citrus fruits, and apples also slow down the production of insulin, so you can eat larger quantities of these without gaining weight. Some high-carb fruits, however, are hands off: watermelon, raisins, pineapples and bananas.

Another important component of this diet is lean meat. The protein in meat stimulates the pancreas to produce glucagon, which, unlike insulin, promotes the breakdown of stored fat. Rather than avoiding steak and eating baked potatoes, as many virtuous dieters do, you should shun the potato and eat the meat instead, according to the authors.

Evidence claimed

Steward and his co-authors look at the long span of human life on earth and focus on the fact that for most of that time, people did not eat refined sugar. No one knew how to refine sugar until about 500 A.D. For the next 1,300 years, refined sugar was relatively rare and usually reserved for the aristocracy, who often developed—not coincidentally, say the authors—obesity, gout, and perhaps diabetes. They claim there is ample evidence to conclude that sugar "just may be the number-one culprit in lowering quality of life and causing premature death." The authors cite a 1976 publication that summarized research on the health hazards of sugar, particularly a worsening incidence of diabetes and other diseases. Graphs of increasing sugar consumption over time suggest a link between this and rising obesity in the United States.

Author Steward, who has been following this diet for five years, avers that he's lost 20 pounds and kept it off. Over 200,000 copies of his originally self-published book have sold in two years, largely, it is claimed, by word of mouth from satisfied dieters. The diet has caught on in New Orleans, a city devoted to good eating and where the obesity rate of 37.5 % is estimated to be the highest in the nation. Every drugstore and corner market peddles the book, and several well-known New Orleans restaurants now offer entrees and desserts that meet this diet's requirements.

The Method

How Sugar Busters! works

Unlike some other diet plans, this program does not specify distinct stages, nor how much weight you can expect to lose. Nor does it tell you how fast the pounds will disappear. The approach is fundamentally simple: You adopt this way of eating and stick with it. The authors do offer a 14-day meal plan to get you started, with lists of acceptable and forbidden foods plus suggested alternatives. They also include 38 pages of mouth-watering recipes from famous New Orleans restaurants featuring oysters, crawfish, steak, shrimp, duck, lamb, and venison, as well as directions on how to make your own whole-wheat pasta.

The authors maintain that eating three meals a day is the way to go, with small, healthy snacks in between. Don't skip meals or you'll change your body's response to insulin and increase fat storage. Beyond that, the diet isn't prescriptive. You don't have to count calories or weigh food—that's just frustrating and unreliable, the authors say. Instead, you concentrate on eating high-fiber carbohydrates, lean meats, and unsaturated fats in appropriate portions. ppropriate means your meat and vegetables should fit on a dinner plate, not hang over the edges. Going back for seconds is a no-no. And no midnight snacks!

What you'll notice

By "virtually eliminating" specified carbohydrates from your diet, say the authors, you'll see your glucose and insulin levels stabilize, your cholesterol drop an average of 15 %, your triglycerides (fatty acids in your blood that have been implicated in heart disease) fall to healthy levels, and your excess pounds vanish. Steward and his co-authors claim that their program will give you an energy surge and improve your health and quality of life. Many people with diabetes, they add, have been weaned off insulin injections after following this diet plan for several years.

Additional steps to take

Other than following the principles of their plan, Steward et al don't mandate any particular steps such as blood tests, visits to the doctor, or nutritional supplements. All the necessary vitamins and minerals are supposedly provided in the foods they promote, so taking supplements is unnecessary. Instead of swallowing a pill, ask the authors, "why not eat a plateful of savory meats and vegetables and lose weight in the process?"

The Diet as Lifestyle

Staying the course

The Sugar Busters! method offers no maintenance program or advice on what to do if you go on a binge or gain back weight you've lost. What if you follow this plan and don't lose weight? The authors cite five common reasons: eating too much of an acceptable carbohydrate such as whole-wheat bread or pasta, too much snacking or too frequent cheating, not exercising, a genetic predisposition to fat storage, or taking hormones such as birth-control pills or menopause supplements, which make it harder to lose weight.

Getting into gear

While the authors do recommend regular, moderate workouts for overall fitness and health, they provide no specific guidelines. One of the authors jokes that the only exercise he gets is when he "lifts his knife and fork." You shouldn't expect to lose much weight with exercise alone, the authors say, especially if you sneak to the pantry and eat forbidden foods.

Evaluating the Diet

Cautions and concerns

Refined sugars are notoriously high in calories, and eliminating them and other readily digested forms of carbohydrates can indeed cause you to lose weight. But as Steward himself admits, the theory behind much of the book's weight-loss strategy is just that: "theoretical." In fact, there's no scientific data to support it. Most people just don't secrete more insulin than they need. If you're normal, your body is a finely tuned sugar-metabolizing machine. Granted, about a quarter of Americans do have chronically elevated amounts of insulin in their blood, the result of a condition called insulin resistance, in which cell receptors for insulin fail to function properly. Many with the syndrome are also overweight. But that doesn't mean those bulges came from eating too much cake. While Sugar Busters! describes obesity as the result of insulin resistance, many experts believe that's putting the cart before the horse. Obesity gives people high insulin, not the other way around.

Calories are not a moot issue. "We are getting fatter," says Gerald Reaven of Stanford University, who years ago was the first researcher to point out the effects of different carbohydrates on blood glucose. "And it is coming from carbohydrates. But the problem isn't the carbohydrates per se; it's that we eat too much of them and take in way too many calories."

Ironically, this diet approach proves Reaven's point. According to a recent analysis, an average day on the plan provides merely 1,200 calories. This may be the book's big secret: It's a low-calorie diet in disguise. Still, there's a downside. Any diet that relies this heavily on meat and full-fat dairy—without being specific about portions—is likely to bring with it a hefty load of artery-clogging saturated fat. (The authors recommend a chocolate mousse, for example, made with five eggs and a quart and a half of heavy cream.) And the wholesale reduction of carbs in your diet will deprive your body of its number one fuel source. No wonder the authors downplay exercise: You likely won't have much energy to work out. Last but not least, when you cut back on certain high-carb fruits and vegetables you may be depriving yourself of essential vitamins and minerals.

Quick fix or lasting results?

When it comes to weight loss there are few shortcuts, even on Bourbon Street. Sugar Busters! doesn't claim you'll lose weight fast, only that you'll lose it permanently if you stick with the program. Since meal plans average only about 1,200 calories daily, most devotees of this diet will take weight off and keep it off—but at a price. Long-term diets below 1,300 calories are generally considered inadequate in nutrients and thus bad for your health.

Flexible or rigid?

If you can give up the proscribed carbohydrates, you'll find the rest of this eating program extremely flexible. You don't have to count calories or measure food in grams, and the authors allow a large variety of meat—even elk, antelope, and alligator! Cheese lovers will find much to admire in this approach: High-fat dairy products are okay.

Stumbling blocks

On the surface, this diet has few stumbling blocks. It's a simplistic, free-wheeling approach to weight loss: Just slash the carbs and you'll lose your extra pounds. Diet on blue-cheese-stuffed filet mignon? No nagging voices ordering you to hit the treadmill? Let the good times roll! But there's potentially serious trouble lurking. Staying on this diet could lead to the biggest stumbling block of all—nutrient deficiency. Without the proper nutrients that a more balanced diet ensures, you could be jeopardizing your health.

Is it for you?

Not if you're a marathon runner or an exercise fanatic, admit the authors, because you need large quantities of glucose to keep you fueled. If you suffer from diabetes, this diet may help control your insulin and glucose levels, though you should check with your doctor before attempting it. Are you an ardent carnivore? Then you'll probably love this diet—just be sure to watch those portions. For Italian food lovers the scenario is bleak, particularly if your grocery store doesn't stock whole-wheat pasta and you don't have time to make your own. Good luck finding pizzas with whole-wheat crust. Vegetarians can skip this one. And for anyone, it's best to think very carefully about whether you really want to follow a program that denies your body its favorite fuel.

Resources

Pick up *Sugar Busters!* (Ballantine, 1998) and its companion, *Sugar Busters! Shopper's Guide*, at your local bookstore. You can visit Sugar Busters! online at www.sugarbusters.com.

The 20/30 Fat
and Fiber Diet Plan

Gabe Mirkin, M.D., author of *Fat Free, Getting Thin* and other bestsellers, appears on a syndicated radio program dealing with issues related to health, fitness, and sexuality. Barry Fox, Ph.D., co-authored the bestseller *The Arthritis Cure*. In *The 20/30 Fat and Fiber Diet Plan*, Mirkin and Fox instruct dieters to limit fats to 20 grams a day and to consume 30 grams of fiber—figures that deviate significantly from most nutritional guidelines. The 20/30 plan, they claim, is a safe, proven, and easy program that has helped thousands lose weight permanently and regain their health.

The Promise

Basic principles of the 20/30 plan

Americans are too heavy because they eat too much fat and too little fiber, the authors contend. By drastically cutting fat intake to 20 grams and increasing dietary fiber to 30 grams a day, they claim you can achieve permanent weight loss without suffering hunger pangs and other unpleasant side effects of dieting. Their approach calls for eating plenty of beans, whole grains, and vegetables. The fat content of their plan is extremely low, and the fiber quite high. For comparison, the USDA says a healthy diet can consist of as much as 30% of calories from fat; on a 2,000-calorie diet, that's about 65 grams. As for fiber, the American Heart Association lists the average daily consumption for Americans at about 15 grams. The 20/30 plan's amount—twice what we typically get—is equivalent to about three cups of canned chickpeas, which are high in fiber, or 10 cups of grated carrots.

The explanation

The authors vow that their low-fat, high-fiber diet will help you shed pounds and keep them off because it's more filling than a high-fat diet, has fewer calories, and consists of foods that take longer to digest. High-fat diets, say Mirkin and Fox, turn people tubby for three reasons: Dietary fat packs more calories per volume than protein or carbohydrates, fat calories are easily converted to body fat, and high-fat low-fiber foods are not filling. On the 20/30 plan, the authors claim, dieters lose weight by eliminating all sources of added fat and any food with more than trace amounts of fat. For most dieters, these changes send calorie consumption into a dive. The bulk of the foods you consume is the secret. "When you eat the same amount of food you've always eaten, but substitute high-fiber foods for the old fatty, low-fiber parts of your diet, you lose weight automatically," say Mirkin and Fox.

> The authors vow that their low-fat, high-fiber diet will help you shed pounds and keep them off because it's more filling.

Evidence claimed

To justify their 20/30 diet plan, the authors refer to a 1997 symposium sponsored by the American Society of Clinical Nutrition, "Fats and Oil Consumption in Health and Disease." The proceedings, published in the American Journal of Clinical Nutrition, reveal a general consensus among nutrition experts from around the world that the most healthful diets concentrate on fruits, vegetables, beans, and whole grains. Mirkin and Fox also provide testimonials from 20/30 plan dieters who have peeled away pounds and kept them off.

The Method

How the 20/30 plan works

On the 20/30 plan you eat no more than 20 grams of fat per day and at least 30 grams of fiber per day. Since a gram of fat produces nine calories (protein and carbohydrates generate only four calories per gram), that's only 180 calories a day—well under 10% of the typical 2,000-calorie diet. Getting your fiber allotment is supposedly easy on this diet: You're encouraged to consume as many fruits, vegetables, beans, and whole grains as you want while limiting refined-flour and other low-fiber foods. You're allowed very sparing amounts of foods such as poultry, whole eggs, beef, pork, and lamb. Most cheeses are limited, unless they're fat-free. Milk and most seafood are off limits. Mirkin and Fox help you jumpstart their plan by providing fat and fiber counts for thousands of foods, including takeout and brand-name items. They also supply hundreds of quick recipes, among them a Southwestern bean dip, an easy-to-prepare chili, and a Sicilian minestrone.

To err, of course, is human, and to accommodate weakness the authors offer the 19 Meals Rule. Each week you follow the 20/30 plan for 19 meals; for the remaining two you eat whatever you want.

What you'll notice

The authors promise that excess pounds will drop away without hunger or the headaches that some dieters suffer, and that you'll begin to glow with health. They give no time frame for when these benefits can be expected, however. They also assert that the program can lower "bad" LDL cholesterol and blood pressure (if it's elevated), slightly raise "good" HDL cholesterol, boost the immune system, and combat diabetes. Furthermore, they say, the 20/30 plan may help impotent men.

Additional steps to take

The authors do not recommend nutritional supplements or medical supervision other than checking with a physician before beginning an exercise program. They do suggest that you drink eight glasses of water a day to avoid dehydration that may result from your increased consumption of fiber.

The Diet as Lifestyle

Staying the course

There are no separate weight-loss and maintenance phases on this diet as there are in many others. From day one you're meant to adopt the 20/30 plan and stick with it for life. Your two free-for-all meals are supposed to stave off the feelings of deprivation that can send your diet into a tailspin.

Getting into gear

Mirkin and Fox recommend 20 to 30 minutes of aerobic activity, such as fast walking, cycling, running, jogging, rollerblading, ice skating, rowing, or aerobic dance. They advise that you do this at least three times a week, along with strength training twice weekly. If you have not been exercising regularly, they strongly suggest that you work up to this level gradually, whether it takes six weeks or six months to get there.

Evaluating the Diet

Cautions and concerns

While 30 grams of fiber a day is a desirable goal, and a high intake of fruits, vegetables, and whole grains is unarguably good for you, the fat allowance on the 20/30 plan is too severe for most people. Keep in mind that this plan calls for 20 grams of fat per day, not 20% of calories from dietary fat. Two tablespoons of butter or a single avocado will put you over the limit, and virtually all types of nuts—except in the most sparing portions—will as well. You'd also have to limit your intake of heart-healthy monounsaturated oils such as olive or canola. But even if you can master such restrictions, keep this in mind: Diets that derive 10% or fewer calories from fat, as this one does for most people, can result in a deficiency of essential fatty acids and the fat-soluble vitamins A, D, E, and K. Basically, the 20-gram rule leaves just enough room for trace amounts of fat in whole grains, fruits, and vegetables.

Another reason to be concerned: Recent studies show that restricting dietary fat to 10% of total calories worsened cholesterol profiles in about a third of healthy men with normal or moderately high cholesterol. Studies by Dr. Ronald Krauss at the University of California at Berkeley suggest that restricting dietary fat causes a shift in LDL cholesterol particles from the normal to the dense, artery-damaging variety. And although Mirkin and Fox claim their diet will cause a slight hike in HDL (the good cholesterol), very-low-fat diets have been shown to lower HDL. Finally, very-low-fat diets are high in carbohydrates, and in some individuals high-carbohydrate diets can elevate triglycerides. While high triglycerides alone normally do not indicate direct risk for heart disease, they do increase risk in people who have other risk factors for cardiovascular disease.

The American Society of Clinical Nutrition symposium that the authors draw on to justify their diet did not, in fact, support the idea that drastic fat restriction improves weight control or overall health. Several presentations at the symposium concluded that a Mediterranean-style diet with its relatively high level of fat, mainly from olive oil, promotes health and longevity. Mediterranean cuisine can also contribute to weight loss. A recent study led by Frank Sacks of the Harvard School of Public Health found that people lose weight just as effectively on a calorie-controlled Mediterranean diet as on a low-fat diet. And in a follow-up study, dieters who were allowed more fat were better able to maintain weight loss. (See the review of *Low-Fat Lies* for more information on the Mediterranean diet.)

Quick fix or lasting results?

The authors promote their 20/30 plan as a lifelong program, not a rapid-results assault on body fat. Of course, drastic reduction of dietary fat will shave off pounds, but the ordeal of consuming 19 no-added-fat meals and only splurging twice a week is likely to weed out all but the most dedicated followers over the long haul. The 20/30 plan might actually work better as a temporary weight-loss regimen; dieters could then ease back into a reasonable higher-fat regimen to keep the weight off.

Flexible or rigid?

The 20/30 plan requires neither calorie counting nor detailed meal plans; it provides built-in calorie control by all but banning dietary fat. And that's the problem: This diet is much too rigid for the average Joe.

Stumbling blocks

Learning to recognize hidden sources of fat so you can cut them from your diet is certainly a practical strategy for weight control. But forbidding even small amounts of unsaturated fat is a tall order. Fat makes food palatable. Dieters who are told that this sort of deprivation is the only way to go may throw up their hands in despair and abandon all effort at weight loss. To tough it out, you'll have to master the art of preparing no-added-fat meals— for example, stir-frying mounds of vegetables with a scant teaspoon of oil. And you may have to cope with howls of protest from family members who don't relish your low-fat feast.

Is it for you?

Not if you have certain health risks, such as high triglycerides, low HDL cholesterol, high blood sugar, or high blood pressure. Regular exercise and a calorie-controlled diet with a moderate amount of mainly monoun-saturated fat would probably be more beneficial for lowering these risk factors for heart disease. Check with your doctor.

If you enjoy the act of eating, you might want to hunt for a more palatable plan. But if you can stomach piles of produce and whole-grain foods while kissing off meat, nuts, avocados, canned tuna, and a myriad other fat-laden foods, you might want to give this diet a try.

Resources

For more on Mirkin and Fox's regimen, pick up *The 20/30 Fat and Fiber Plan (Harper Collins 2000)* at your local bookstore, or log on to www.2030plan.com.

Volumetrics: Feeling Full on Fewer Calories

Barbara Rolls, Ph.D., a nutrition researcher at Pennsylvania State University, and Robert Barnett, a journalist who writes about food and nutrition, join forces to present a weight-control program based on "the science of satiety." In *Volumetrics: Feeling Full on Fewer Calories,* the authors argue that it's the volume of food you eat, not the number of calories, that makes you feel full. Rolls has been researching hunger and obesity for more than 20 years, during which time she served as president of the North American Association for the Study of Obesity. She has also served on the advisory council of the National Institutes of Health's Institute of Diabetes and Digestion and Kidney Diseases. Her years of research, she says, support her contention that if you know the secrets of satiety, you won't feel hungry when you cut back on calories.

The Promise

Basic principles of Volumetrics

The key to controlling weight is no great mystery: You have to create a calorie deficit, burning more than you consume either by eating less, using more, or both. Rolls and Barnett say the easiest way to achieve a calorie deficit is to reduce the number of calories you eat each day. But cutting calories, they claim, doesn't mean you'll have to don the hair shirt of hunger and deprivation—at least not if you make smart food choices. Learn which foods fill you up on fewer calories and make those the centerpiece of your menu, the authors promise, and you'll control your weight without ever thinking diet.

> The key to controlling weight is no great mystery: You have to create a calorie deficit, burning more than you consume.

The explanation

According to Rolls and Barnett, we tend to eat the same average weight in food from day to day regardless of the number of calories we take in. It stands to reason, the authors contend, that if you eat the same weight of food but lower the calories, you'll shave pounds without hunger. So how do you reduce calories without shrinking portions? "Dilute" your meals, say the authors. Choose low-cal, high-volume foods that have lots of water or fiber (both of which promote satiety) such as fruit, vegetables, low-fat milk, and lean meat, and go easy on high-cal, low-volume foods such as nuts, cheese, and crackers, as well as candy and low-fat cookies. You have to eat a lot of those high-calorie, or energy-dense, foods before you feel full, and that packs on the pounds. "Low-energy-dense" foods fill you up without the extra calorie load.

Evidence claimed

To support their theories, Rolls and Barnett refer to numerous studies into the relationship between food, hunger, and satiety—many performed at reputable institutions such as the National Institutes of Health. The authors rely most on research done at Penn State's Laboratory for the Study of Human Ingestive Behavior, of which Rolls is the director. In one study at Penn State, normal-weight women were served all their meals and snacks in the lab over three two-day periods. They were allowed to eat as much of the main course—which varied in energy density from day to day—as they liked. No matter what the energy density of the food, the women all ate about the same weight of food each day, roughly three pounds total. On days when low-energy-density meals were served, they ate about 400 fewer calories but felt just as full and satisfied, suggesting that calories don't matter when it comes to satiety.

Despite such research, the authors admit, the study of calorie density and its influence on the human appetite is still relatively new. Long-term studies of the effectiveness of their approach to weight management are few, though clinical trials are in the works. But Rolls and Barnett do note that Roland L. Weinsier, a professor at the University of Alabama, has for 25 years run a weight-loss program based on a low-fat, low-energy-dense diet with good results.

The Method

How Volumetrics works

The program is based on a simple formula for determining how many calories you need each day. You multiply your weight by a certain number depending on whether you're male or female, sedentary or active: If you're a sedentary woman, multiply by 12;

an active woman, multiply by 14; a sedentary man, 15; and an active man, 17. Now, to achieve weight loss at a reasonable rate of one pound a week, subtract 500 from the number you got. That's how many calories you should consume daily. Once you've achieved significant weight loss—say, 12 pounds in 12 weeks—your calorie needs will have changed and you'll need to rework the formula based on your new weight if you still need to lose. The program's weight-loss phase should last no more than six months, at which point you switch to a maintenance plan.

The program is based on a simple formula for determining how many calories you need each day.

Rolls and Barnett provide daily menu plans to help you put the weight-loss portion of the program into practice. These are based on either a 1,600- or a 2,000-calorie diet; you fine-tune the calorie level to your own target by adding or subtracting suggested snacks. The 1,600-calorie plan calls for a 400-calorie breakfast, a 500-calorie lunch, a 500-calorie dinner, and a snack or dessert of 200 calories. The 2,000-calorie plan is similar but adds more calories at each meal. The menu plan is modular, so that each day you can choose whichever combination of breakfast, lunch, dinner, and snack you want from a list of options. The list includes 12 breakfast ideas, 10 lunches, 25 dinners, and dozens of snacks.

Rolls and Barnett also offer guidelines for dieters who want to plan their own meals. Some 20 to 30% of your total calories should come from fat, 55 % or more should come from carbohydrates (primarily whole grains, vegetables, and fruits), and about 15 % should come from protein. These figures mirror those recommended by the USDA and many nutritionists. Low-energy-dense protein choices include beans, low-fat fish, poultry without the skin, and lean meat. In addition, the authors say, you should aim for 20 to 30 grams of fiber a day to lower the calorie density of meals and to satisfy hunger—again, figures that jibe with the USDA recommendation. You should also go easy on added sugars, especially sugary drinks, which jack up calories without doing much to alleviate hunger. But you don't have to give up your favorite foods or alter your diet completely. Some calorie-dense foods like nuts, the authors say, are very nutritious, and others, like chocolate, are "too delicious to give up."

To help you distinguish low-energy- from high-energy-dense foods, Volumetrics supplies calorie densities for more than 600 foods. The book also offers a variety of recipes for low-energy-dense appetizers, soups (promoted heavily in the book as excellent appetite quenchers), salads, entrees, desserts, blender drinks, and breakfasts.

What you'll notice

If you stick to their plan, Rolls and Barnett say, you'll prune calories without feeling deprived, and some people, they claim, may actually have to get used to eating more food rather than less. The authors also maintain that you'll enjoy better health from the outset—even before casting off fat—because their plan is nutritionally balanced and heart healthy.

Additional steps to take

In addition to eating water-packed foods like tomatoes, you should drink lots of water during the day, say the authors. Between "straight" water and the water in foods, women should get about nine cups a day, and men about 12. If alcohol is part of your diet, make sure you don't consume more than a drink a day if you're a woman and two per day if you're a man.

Rolls and Barnett also recommend that you keep food and exercise logs. In the food log, you'll record what you eat at each meal and snack, serving sizes, and your feelings as you go through the day. You can refer to this log to help you determine where to substitute high- with low-energy-dense foods. During the weight-loss phase, the authors counsel, you should step on the scale au naturel once a week at the same hour. During maintenance, you may want to weigh yourself more frequently so as to counter moderate wieght gains before they balloon out of control.

The Diet as Lifestyle

Staying the course

The authors deal directly with the problem of falling off the diet wagon. You had a doughnut on your way into work this morning. Should you write off the day as a lost cause and eat whatever you like until tomorrow? No way, say Rolls and Barnett. You can salvage the slip with smart choices at lunch and dinner. But don't try to compensate by skipping meals or slashing calories; you might get stuck in a binge-and-starve rut. If temptation is looming on the horizon—an upcoming party or other social occasion—plan a self-control strategy, and then if you manage to stick with it, reward yourself with a nonfood treat.

After six months you should switch to the maintenance plan even if you haven't reached your weight goal, advise Rolls and Barnett. Guidelines for maintenance are similar to those for weight loss; the only difference is you're allowed more calories each day. Once you've maintained your weight for six months, if you still have more to lose you're to go back to the weight-loss program. According to the authors, after maintaining your weight goal within a five-pound range for two years, you're a winner.

Getting into gear

Exercise is crucial, especially for maintaining weight loss. Why? As Rolls and Barnett explain it, when you reduce calories to lose weight, you're shedding not only fat but also lean body mass—in other words, muscle. This isn't desirable because a pound of muscle burns more calories than a pound of body fat, even at rest. But exercise builds muscle, increasing your resting metabolic rate. Furthermore, you burn lots of calories while exercising and keep burning them for several hours afterward. Just as important, exercise helps you stay committed to a healthier lifestyle by "boosting your mood, lowering anxiety, curbing depression, improving sleep, and improving your sense of self-esteem." And exercise brings with it a cascade of health benefits, including a reduced risk of heart attack and stroke.

The authors recommend that you engage in moderate exercise for at least 30 minutes most days, if not every day. Walking at a pace of three to four miles per hour is ideal for most people. To make your exercise more effective, you should periodically lengthen the workout or increase its intensity. And twice a week you should include some resistance training. Your exercise log will help you keep track of when you need to make changes.

Evaluating the Diet

Cautions and concerns

There really isn't much to criticize in the Volumetrics approach. Its recommended percentages of calories derived from protein, fat, and carbohydrate echo those of the American Heart Association, and the emphasis on vegetables and fruit, limited saturated fat, and balance in the diet reflect the basic principles underlying the USDA Food Guide Pyramid (see "A Guide to Good Dieting" at the front of this book). Rolls and Barnett encourage you to eat a healthy variety of produce, pasta, whole grains, soups, low-fat dairy, seafood, and lean poultry and meat. While much of the research used to support this diet is new and long-term results are unavailable, the plan promotes healthy eating habits and represents a sensible approach to dieting.

Quick fix or lasting results?

This is no quick fix, but there's nothing wrong with that. The authors recommend safe, gradual weight loss through the creation of a mild calorie deficit. "It's a lifestyle plan, not a diet," they say. The authors contend that the Volumetrics philosophy is the basis for other successful weight-management programs, including Weight Watchers' 1•2•3 Success® plan (see the reviews of that plan and of *Dieting with the Duchess*).

Flexible or rigid?

On the Volumetrics plan, you're encouraged to eat a wide variety of foods. Better yet, you don't have to give up all your favorites—not even chocolate. And so long as you stay within the calorie corral, you can put together menus to suit your tastes. Still, you'd better have a hankering for fruit, vegetables, soup, and other low-energy-dense options. Suggested recipes and meal plans are ideal for all members of the family.

Stumbling blocks

There's not much to stand in your way of making this approach work. You do have to make some calculations, and there are a few complex formulas for determining just how overweight you are. To determine the energy density of a food, you'll have to read the nutrition label and divide the number of calories by the number of grams per serving. One potential stumbling block: The plan's very flexibility—no banned foods—could be a dieter's excuse to overindulge in sinfully delicious, high-cal treats. You'll need to exercise some common sense.

Is it for you?

This program teaches the sort of healthy eating habits that can ease you toward your ideal weight and keep you there, so if you want to melt fat in a matter of weeks, look elsewhere. Volumetrics serves up lots of health-wise advice—a welcome change from diet books that sound as if they're written by used-car salesmen, full of fast talk and empty promises. Rolls and Barnett also caution that if you're overeating for emotional reasons such as depression, their weight control plan won't help until you've addressed that issue first.

Resources

Rolls and Barnett's *Volumetrics: Feel Full on Fewer Calories* is published by HarperCollins (2000). A resource guide in the back of the book lists helpful sources of information on weight control, including websites.

Weight Watchers'
1·2·3 Success® Plan

Weight Watchers, a commercial weight-loss program, was founded in 1963 when Jean Nidetch gathered friends in her Brooklyn home to begin brainstorming about how to shed unwanted pounds. Since then, the program claims, it has helped more than 25 million people worldwide. According to Weight Watchers' own statistics, the current version of the program, 1·2·3 Success®, is the most successful yet, having guided almost four million people to their weight-loss goals in North America alone. For a fee, Weight Watchers helps you track calories without severely curbing menu choices. But what really distinguishes this approach from the vast majority of weight-loss plans is support. Weekly group meetings teach you healthy eating and exercise habits and let you share your dieting ups and downs—and learn from those of others.

The Promise

Basic principles of the Weight Watchers approach

When you join Weight Watchers, the program pledges to help you shed weight safely and effectively by providing guidance and inspiration. Staff members—everyone from leaders to receptionists—have all participated in the Weight Watchers program and undergo regular training to keep current. You'll receive resources teaching you how to reduce caloric intake without eliminating the foods you love. This is basically a low-calorie, high-fiber diet that promotes exercise and other healthy changes in your lifestyle. Recognizing that dieting is more than just physical, the program also addresses the issue of psychological obstacles to weight loss.

The explanation

The 1·2·3 Success plan assigns foods a point value based on calorie, fat, and fiber content. You're allotted a specific range of total points each day that's based on your current body weight and your weight goal; a range of 22 to 29 points is typical. You can "spend" that total however you like. If you want to blow your entire day's allotment on hot fudge sundaes with whipped cream, that's okay. But of course you're encouraged to distribute your points more wisely, across a wider variety of foods. You can buy packaged foods tagged with Weight Watchers point values at the grocery store, though you don't have to do so in order to keep with the program; printed guides indicate the points assigned to more than 12,000 popular food items, and any edible not on the list can be assigned points as long as you know its calorie, fat, and fiber content. The point system allows you to keep eating the foods you like without exceeding the calorie limit deemed appropriate for your weight goal. Diets range from 1,225 to 1,745 calories per day.

This is basically a low-calorie, high-fiber diet that promotes exercise and other healthy changes in your lifestyle.

Evidence claimed

The Weight Watchers International Scientific Council includes registered dieticians, exercise physiologists, and clinical psychologists. "In addition to our staff of professionals," says Weight Watchers promotional literature, "we regularly consult with experts from around the world who are on the cutting edge of the latest scientific discoveries. Rest assured that we work diligently to incorporate the best that medical science has to offer into our program." The literature is also full of inspirational testimonials but provides little in the way of specific scientific evidence demonstrating the efficacy of the program.

Weight Watchers' lead scientist, Karen Miller-Kovach, rejects fad diets as nutritionally unbalanced, ineffective for long-term weight loss, and scientifically unproven. Instead, she recommends the Weight Watchers approach of a quality diet, moderate portions, plenty of exercise—and the buddy system. The Weight Watchers website refers to a university study demonstrating that "dieters who recruited three friends or family members to support them in their quest had better results losing weight and keeping it off than did dieters who had no buddy system to fall back on." Promotional literature cites a recent study suggesting that followers of the Weight Watchers approach achieve more satisfying results than people who try to lose weight on their own. The literature also refers to unnamed scientific studies showing that even a modest weight loss of 10%—the first step of the 1·2·3 Success program—helps lower the health risks associated with obesity.

The Method

How the Weight Watchers approach works

According to Weight Watchers, the best way to achieve weight loss is step by small step. The first stage is the so-called "10% difference™," during which you shed 5 to 10% of your current weight. Once your belt loosens, says Weight Watchers, you'll be motivated to enter two more stages, first "feel the difference," and then "live the difference."

Weight Watchers makes no guarantees about how quickly you'll reach your target weight, and the literature is careful to point out that individuals lose weight at different rates, depending on age, gender, current weight, and commitment to the program. Rapid weight loss, Weight Watchers warns, is dangerous to your health and usually not sustainable. In general, the program is designed for a loss of up to two pounds a week, except in the beginning when you might lose more easily. If you happen to lose weight faster, you'll be urged to slow down.

The staff at Weight Watchers will help you figure out your weight goals and will arm you with battle plans to achieve those goals. But ultimately, the responsibility lies with you. You stay on the program as long as you like, depending on how much weight you want to lose and how faithful you are to the program.

What you'll notice

According to one testimonial, on the Weight Watchers plan you'll improve your health and have "increased energy, sharper focus, and even the simple joy of better-fitting clothes." Casting off 10% of your weight, you're assured, will send your confidence soaring and strengthen your motivation to lose more.

Additional steps to take

There's much more to Weight Watchers than cutting calories. If points and percentages are the heart of Weight Watchers, then group support is its soul. Every week you're supposed to attend a confidential weigh-in and pay a weekly fee (there's also a registration fee). Once the weekly fee is paid you can attend as many group meetings as you like that week—and you're urged to attend at least one. At meetings, experienced leaders dispense nutritional advice and serve as role models, helping you tackle obstacles, cheering you on, and celebrating your successes.

Upon joining the program, you'll receive the Weight Watchers Tools for Living, a set of techniques to help you cope with the thoughts and feelings that can derail your weight-loss plans. Techniques include "reframing," a way of replacing negative behavior with positive, and mental rehearsing, in which you envision yourself saying no to temptation.

Weight Watchers encourages you to consult with your physician before starting the program. You're advised to have periodic check-ups and to take vitamin and mineral supplements, which are available through Weight Watchers (as are Weight Watchers food products).

The Diet as Lifestyle

Staying the course

After you've passed through the first two stages, you enter the stage called "live the difference." Weight Watchers teaches you how to shift from the mindset of weight loss to one of weight control. This is a tricky time, when old eating habits beckon and threaten to waylay you. It's recommended that you continue to attend meetings for at least six weeks after reaching your weight goal.

Once you've remained within two pounds of your goal for six consecutive weeks, and you weigh at least five pounds less than when you started the program, you're eligible for Weight Watchers Lifetime Membership. As a lifetime member you pay no fees, but you have to weigh in once each calendar month at no more than two pounds over your goal weight. An added plus of lifetime membership: You can apply for a job with Weight Watchers.

Getting into gear

There is no elevator to success; you have to take the stairs. This saying could be Weight Watchers' motto. The program includes another points system designed to help you find the level of physical activity that's appropriate for you; it involves a simple formula that factors in your weight, the intensity of the activity, and time. Activity points earn you additional food points—that is, the more you exercise, the more you're allowed to eat. Weight Watchers encourages aerobic workouts and resistance training, but if you're the type who prefers gardening to gyms, that's fine. The idea is to make exercise an integral part of your weight-loss and maintenance program.

Evaluating the Diet

Cautions and concerns

If you abide by Weight Watchers' nutritional recommendations and point system, this program should help you lose weight safely. It combines calorie cutbacks with exercise, which is what most nutrition experts recommend, and although it gives you the freedom to eat as you like, it also encourages healthful food choices. The support system may also prove invaluable to you in your efforts. One cautionary note: Some of Weight Watchers' own food products contain additives that are deemed unhealthy by some nutritionists. Also, keep in mind that this is not a medically supervised program. If you're extremely overweight or have medical conditions associated with obesity, see a doctor before joining this program.

Despite the group cheerleading, whether this plan will work for you depends very much on your own efforts. Although the point system encourages you to make diet-smart choices—foods with the fewest points are scant in calories and fat, high in healthful fiber—it's up to you to eat a varied diet with a nutritious balance of carbohydrates, fats, and proteins. When it comes to weight loss and healthy eating, ultimately you're on your own.

Quick fix or lasting results?

This isn't just a program—it's a way of life. According to a Weight Watchers survey, about half the program's lifetime members maintained their weight loss after two years. No information is offered about this survey or its accuracy. Given Weight Watchers' sensible overall approach, however—not least, the recommendation that you follow a balanced diet, which, given the human appetite for variety, is the surest way to stave off food cravings—such encouraging results seem entirely possible.

Flexible or rigid?

Weight Watchers' ingenious point system takes the guesswork out of calorie, fiber, and fat tallying. No foods to weigh, no calories to count, no labels to pore over. You don't even have to purchase Weight Watchers. The

1·2·3 Success plan gives you the freedom to consume whatever foods you fancy. On top of it all, there are thousands of convenient meeting locations to choose from. If you can't escape the office, Weight Watchers will set up an at-work program for you and your co-workers. And if you dread group meetings, you might be eligible, depending on where you live, for an at-home version of the program.

Stumbling blocks

You might just balk at the financial commitment that the Weight Watchers program involves. Be prepared to shell out when you climb on board and every time you weigh in. The one-time registration fee is typically $16 to $20, the weekly fee $10 to $15, whether you're in weight loss or maintenance. If you miss six consecutive weeks your membership is discontinued, though you can re-register at any time. Since you don't know how long you'll be in Weight Watchers, there's no way to determine the total cost—something to keep in mind if your budget's tight. Moreover, you'll have to bring your membership book to every weigh-in as proof that you're a bona fide, paid-up weight watcher.

Note that while you may not be counting calories, you'll still be adding up points. Weight Watchers claims that its points system is easy, but not all foods are included on the list. To determine point values for unlisted foods, you'll have to scrape together fat, fiber, and calorie figures and plug them into a formula.

Is it for you?

If you shudder at the thought of people keeping an eye on your dieting struggles, or if you're turned off by support group settings, this program isn't for you. Men who feel uncomfortable when they're in the minority might also want to think twice: Weight Watchers groups are overwhelmingly female.

Special adaptations of the program are available for nursing mothers and teens. Kids under 10 must have permission from a physician to participate. The program doesn't accept pregnant women, people suffering from bulimia nervosa, or individuals whose weight is less than five pounds above the minimum set out in the Weight Watchers weight range. If you have a medical condition or are on a prescription drug, or if you're grossly overweight, consult with a physician before joining this program.

Resources

W eight Watchers is headquartered at 175 Crossways Park West, Woodbury, NY 11797. The program offers various motivational aids designed to help you control your weight (even if you aren't a member), including cookbooks, exercise videos, audiocassette tapes and books such as *Weight Stages: Successfully Manage Your Weight Through Life's Ups and Downs*. See also the review of *Dieting with the Duchess*. For more information about Weight Watchers or to join the program, call 800-651-6000 or log on to www.weightwatchers.com.

Eating Well for Optimum Health: The Essential Guide to Food, Diet, and Nutrition

Andrew Weil's take on the ideal diet can be summarized in two words: balance and variety. This Harvard-trained physician who directs the program in integrative medicine at the University of Arizona shuns low-carb and low-fat regimens as well as nondairy vegetarian (vegan) diets. The best approach to eating, says this proponent of holistic medicine, draws on all three macronutrients—carbohydrate, fat, and protein. Eating an abundance of fresh fruits and vegetables and avoiding processed foods, says Weil, will meet your nutritional needs while fortifying your body against disease. The emphasis here is less on weight loss than on living a long and healthy life.

The Promise

Basic principles of the Eating Well approach

Confusing, contradictory information about diet and nutrition bombards the public daily. To set the record straight, Weil aims to educate you about what your body really does with the foods you feed it. The best diet performs four basic tasks. First, it gives you all the calories, macronutrients, and micronutrients you need to function. Second, it increases your chance of a long life by fortifying your body's defenses and natural healing mechanisms. Third, it makes eating a pleasurable experience, not an exercise in self-denial. And finally, it encourages social interaction and includes foods that express your personal or cultural identity. Eating well, Weil contends, is as important to the spirit as it is to the body.

If your goal is to lose weight, you'll need to exercise more and eat less—how much less Weil doesn't say. But being overweight isn't necessarily unhealthy, adds Weil. He draws a line between people who are active and fit in spite carrying extra pounds, and those who are "morbidly obese"—whose extra weight compromises their health and longevity.

The explanation

As you spin your cart through the grocery store, what foods should you leave on the shelf? Some diet gurus weigh in against carbohydrates. Others tell you fat is the enemy. Who's right? Weil guides you through this culinary conundrum, beginning with a scientific treatise on macronutrients (carbohydrates, fats, and proteins) and micronutrients (vitamins, minerals, fiber, and phytochemicals). On his list of foods to embrace: wild salmon, walnuts, and other foods rich in omega-3 essential fatty acids (these help make cell membranes flexible and are found in hormones that prevent abnormal blood clotting and inflammation); extra-virgin olive oil (high in monounsaturated fat and low in trans-fatty acids, the fats that interfere with the formation of healthy cell membranes and hormones); soy products (rich in protein, omega-3s, and isoflavones—phytochemicals that may help protect against some forms of cancer); and a wide variety of fruits and vegetables (preferably organic because, Weil claims, organic produce is richer in nutrients). Topping his list of foods to shun: processed foods made with refined white flour such as pastries and white bread (low in fiber and usually high in fat); polyunsaturated oils including safflower, sunflower, sesame, corn, soy, and cottonseed oils (they can oxidize into possible-cancer-promoting compounds that are also harmful to the cardiovascular system); deep-fried products, especially from fast-food restaurants (reheated oil may be toxic); and foods made with partially hydrogenated oil, which is full of trans-fatty acids.

Less scientifically, Weil subscribes to the belief that food conveys "a form of vital energy that we need or even the emotional and spiritual vibrations of the people who have handled it." He touts the benefits of organic produce, arguing that it packs more nutrients and more vital energy than conventionally grown produce. The cook who prepares a meal with loving care transfers that positive energy to the food, says Weil. The same meal prepared by an angry, resentful cook passes on negative emotional energy.

Evidence claimed

Weil has spent years studying the medical literature on nutrition and working with patients to improve their diets. To back up his belief in the significance of diet to your health and longevity, he relies on studies that look at large populations. For example, he mentions the dip in deaths from heart attacks in Denmark, Holland,

and other occupied countries during World War II when popular foods such as butter, cheese, and meat were scarce. Once this saturated-fat-laden fare reappeared, the incidence of heart attacks rebounded. As evidence of another danger of the typical Western diet, Weil points to a study of Japanese women. They have one of the lowest rates of breast cancer worldwide, yet when they move to the United States and adopt its diet, their risk of getting this disease rises sharply. And as the Western diet infiltrates China and Japan, those countries are experiencing a rise in the rate of typically Western conditions such as heart disease.

Weil's book is packed with references to scientific studies and surveys, and to his credit he doesn't distort their results to prove his theories. Whenever he makes a claim for which there is no scientific evidence—such as the notion that food contains the "spiritual vibrations of the people who have handled it"— Weil is the first to admit it.

The Method

How the Eating Well approach works

Weil's dietary program involves no stages or funky meal schedules. In general, he recommends that you consume between 2,000 and 3,000 calories a day depending on your gender, your body size, and how physically active you are. Of these calories, 50 to 60% should come from carbohydrate, 30% from fat, and 10 to 20% from protein—the standard breakdown recommended by mainstream nutritionists. When choosing carbohydrates, Weil advises, limit refined, processed foods with a high glycemic index (foods that convert quickly to glucose during digestion). Foods with a low glycemic index such as whole grains, carrots, beans, and many nontropical fruits help slow down the absorption of glucose and should be included in every meal. When choosing fats, he counsels, you should aim for a ratio of 1:2:1 for saturated to monounsaturated to polyunsaturated. You're best off eating less full-fat dairy such as cheese, butter, and cream, fatty meats, and unskinned chicken, avoiding margarine, vegetable shortening, products made with partially hydrogenated oils and all deep-fried chow, and—to get healthy omega-3 fatty acids—consuming more oily fish, fortified eggs, soybeans, and walnuts. Protein should come primarily from vegetables such as beans, says Weil, but may also come from fish and reduced-fat dairy products. If you have a liver or kidney condition, allergies, or autoimmune problems, you should reduce your intake of protein altogether. Eating more fruits, vegetables, and whole grains will give a healthy lift to the amount of fiber in your system—and eating a variety of these foods along with mushrooms, says Weil, will help protect you from cancer, degenerative disease, and environmental toxins.

Want to lose weight? Weil advises cutting calories across the board.

Want to lose weight? Weil advises cutting calories across the board, maintaining a healthy balance of macronutrients but reducing portions at meals and snacks. Meals should leave you feeling satisfied, not cheated. Weil includes a chapter with dozens of healthy recipes to get you started.

What you'll notice

A healthy diet," Weil teaches, "is the cornerstone of a healthy lifestyle." And it brings a cascade of benefits, if you believe the first-hand accounts sprinkled throughout this book from Weil converts. What you may notice, following his path, is a steadier emotional life, greater energy, weight loss, and more control over chronic conditions such as asthma, allergies, and arthritis. You may even find dietary cures for common ailments ranging from athlete's foot to sinus problems. Food choices can serve a battery of medicinal purposes, believes Weil, who dispenses dietary advice to cope with common ailments.

Additional steps to take

To wise up about nutrients, says Weil, you should become adept at the art of reading food labels. Under his tutelage you'll become a veritable food-label detective, learning how to sniff out harmful chemicals and pump up your intake of healing nutrients. Weil also recommends that you take an array of supplements to meet your full nutritional needs, including vitamins C and E, the B-complex vitamins, selenium, carotenoids, and calcium. You should also drink six to eight glasses of water a day as well as a cup or two of tea, especially green tea, for the antioxidants it contains. (Antioxidants are compounds that battle free radicals, molecules that may injure cell membranes, enzymes, and DNA.)

The Diet as Lifestyle

Staying the course

Weil isn't a martinet—there's no one right way to eat, he says, and because our nutritional needs tend to change over time, no diet is set in concrete. As time goes by, you should keep abreast of your body's changing needs and adjust your dietary choices. If you're gaining weight, he advises, increase your physical activity, eat smaller portions and snack less often. Every bit you do to improve your eating habits is reason for self-congratulation; don't waste time chastising yourself for the occasional binge on French fries or potato chips.

Getting into gear

When it comes to losing weight, Weil has some straightforward advice: Get moving. To shed pounds you've got to cut down on calories and burn more calories through physical activity. Exercise, says Weil, burns calories in the short term and also alters your body's "set point" for weight and appetite, which helps you lose weight and keep it off down the road. Intense workouts at the gym are fine, if that's your bag, but you're just as well off, says Weil, if you simply make an effort to be more active throughout the day, climbing stairs, walking, gardening, doing housework, anything that gets you in gear.

Evaluating the Diet

Cautions and concerns

Weil's basic principles—in recommended percentages of fat, protein, and carbohydrate—parallel those of most respected nutritional programs, including that of the American Heart Association. And his notions about variety and balance in food choice reflect the central premise of the USDA Food Guide Pyramid (see "A Guide to Good Dieting" at the front of this book). This is no outlandish get-thin-quick plan. If you follow Weil's advice, you'll be deporting junk food from your pantry and meeting your daily nutritional needs.

Which isn't to say you'll lose weight. Weil's distinction between those who are physically fit in spite of being overweight and those who are "morbidly obese" may be a pitfall for would-be weight losers. Weil argues that Western culture's fat-phobia has influenced the medical community to overstate the health risks of excess bulk. As long as you keep fit and maintain a healthy diet, he suggests, you can ignore the obsession with poundage and live a long and healthy life. This observation is refreshing insofar as it encourages overweight people not to hate their bodies. The problem is, no specific guidelines are given for determining which category you fall into. Skating on Weil's thin ice of commentary, the morbidly obese may succumb to the wishful belief that they rank among the ordinary overweight and ignore medical advice. That could be a fatal mistake, since obesity raises the risk of diabetes, heart disease, stroke, and other health problems, and each year causes tens or even hundreds of thousands of premature deaths in the United States. Would-be weight losers won't find specific guidelines on daily caloric intake in these pages. If you stick with the 2,000- to 3,000-calorie range Weil recommends for a healthy diet, you could end up gaining rather than losing weight.

Quick fix or lasting results?

Weil's optimum diet is a lifetime philosophy of eating, not a slam-bang weight-loss plan. It aims to increase your chances of a long and healthy life. There is little hard evidence to support the efficacy of his approach, however. Weil includes success stories to inspire a sea change in your eating habits, but no hard facts indicating how many people have adopted his approach or how it improved their health.

Flexible or rigid?

As long as you can bear to ban junk food and cut down on almost all fats except olive oil and the omega-3 fatty acids found in salmon and sardines, you'll find plenty of leeway in this diet. That's because Weil encourages you to apply his principles to an eating style that suits you. You'll need to keep an eye on the ratio of carbs, proteins, and fats in your diet, differentiate between high- and low-glycemic carbs, watch the proportions of different kinds of fat, and tally calories for a week to see whether you're overloading on certain foods. But with a little practice, the arithmetic of ratios and calories should become second nature.

Stumbling blocks

Watch out for your wallet—one of the potential pitfalls with Weil's approach is financial. Dieters who follow his plan load up on a wide variety of organic produce, which can be expensive. Nonvegetarians are instructed to purchase hormone- and drug-free meat and poultry—generally higher-ticket items—as well as wild salmon, which is three to four times as costly as the farm-raised variety. An additional drain on the dollars: a preference for extra virgin olive oil over all other fats—even canola oil, which most nutritionists okay.

As for digesting the fine print on food labels, this could turn the already-time-consuming activity of grocery shopping into a marathon. Plus, you'll be spending lots of extra time preparing meals to avoid processed foods—a potential stumbling block for some.

Is it for you?

If you're ready to shed pounds quickly, this program may disappoint. The focus of Weil's program is eating for health, not to lose weight. But Weil's approach isn't to be dismissed lightly. This well-trained physician offers an approach to good nutrition that reinforces the principles of balance and variety advocated by most mainstream nutrition experts. If you adopt his approach, cut back on your usual portions, and exercise regularly, you'll probably lose weight over the long term without compromising your health. A vegetarian himself, Weil addresses the concerns of non-meat eaters while giving carnivores space to indulge. Only vegans—vegetarians who bar diary products and fish—need skip this diet. Dairy products and fish are too critical to your health to be banned from the diet, says Weil.

Resources

For details, check out *Eating Well for Optimum Health: The Essential Guide to Food, Diet, and Nutrition* (Alfred A. Knopf, 2000). You can find additional information about dieting and nutrition, and subscribe to Dr. Andrew Weil's *Self Healing Newsletter,* a monthly publication with up-to-date information about natural healing, by logging on to www.drweil.com.

The Zone

In this best-selling book Barry Sears—a medical researcher who has invented delivery systems for drugs used in treating cancer and heart disease—applies his biotechnology experience to the subject of dieting. Sears and coauthor Bill Lawren challenge dieters to think of food not as a source of pleasure or a means of satisfying hunger but rather as a powerful drug. According to Sears, food administered in precise amounts at specific times can alter your hormonal balance and send you into a near-euphoric state called the Zone, where weight loss is almost automatic, your mind is sharp yet relaxed, and your muscles work like a well-oiled machine. Sears has designed a "dietary road map" that he claims will direct you into the Zone and keep you there.

The Promise

Basic principles of the Zone diet

Although Americans are eating less fat, says Sears, obesity is on the rise; between 1980 and 1991, it increased by a staggering 32 %. What's the problem? According to Sears, it's that we're eating more carbohydrates than ever before. Carbohydrates are found in bread, pasta, candy, dairy products, fruit, and vegetables. Your body, Sears maintains, can store only a limited amount of carbohydrate; when you eat too much at one meal—even the carbohydrates in fat-free rice cakes—your body converts the excess into body fat. To enter the zone of permanent weight loss and peak health, Sears contends, you should eat food "in a controlled fashion and in the proper proportions—as if it were an intravenous drip." That means reducing your intake of carbs to about 40% of total calories (the USDA recommends 60%), making up the loss by doubling the standard protein amount to 30%, and getting 30% from fat (the USDA maximum), most of which should be monounsaturated. Sears calls this the 40-30-30 diet. If you lopped off the base of the USDA Food Pyramid, he notes, you'd have a zone-favorable diet. (See "A Guide to Good Dieting" at the front of this book for more information on the food pyramid.)

The explanation

Like other advocates of low-carbohydrate dieting (see "A Guide to Good Dieting" for the complete list), Sears begins with some generally accepted information about how the body metabolizes food to create energy. Carbohydrates—a class of carbon-based compounds that includes sugars, starch, and cellulose—are the body's main source of fuel. When you eat carbs, your digestive system breaks them down into glucose, a form of sugar, which enters your bloodstream. In response, your pancreas secretes the hormone insulin, whose job it is to convert glucose into energy for the use of your body's cells. When there is more glucose than the body can use for energy, insulin converts the excess into stored fat. And that's the problem with insulin, says Sears, that it tells your body to store fat and keep it stored. Sears's conclusion: The more carbs you eat, the harder it is to lose weight. According to the author, 75 % of us will fail on a high-carb diet because elevated insulin levels cause us to accumulate body fat. He says the worst carbs are the ones that rate very high on the glycemic index, a measure of how fast a carbohydrate is broken down into glucose. Foods that break down quickly—the so-called simple carbohydrates such as table sugar and honey, as well as breads and pasta—drive your blood sugar and therefore insulin levels up, turning your body into a fat producer.

According to Sears, his diet works because it mimics the diet of our hunting and gathering ancestors.

Sears's logic also depends on other information about metabolism. Whenever you eat macronutrients—carbohydrate, dietary fat, and protein—you set in motion a complex series of hormonal responses. As Sears explains it, carbs stimulate the production of insulin, which reduces blood sugar levels, but protein has an opposite effect: It causes the pancreas to release the hormone glucagon, which increases blood sugar levels by releasing stored carbohydrates from the liver. Properly balanced glucagon and insulin levels open the portal to the Zone, Sears asserts. As for dietary fat, he goes on, it supplies you with essential fatty acids, which form the building blocks of the so-called superhormones, the eicosanoids. The author asserts that eicosanoids are the chemical moderators that supervise all the body's hormonal reactions. Achieving your ideal protein-to-carb ratio will help you balance your "good" and "bad" eicosanoids, he says. Supposedly, bad eicosanoids ratchet up insulin production, while good ones allay hunger. Furthermore, Sears maintains, the eicosanoids control the release of stored body fat. To lose fat, says the author, you have to eat fat.

Evidence claimed

Sears says his diet is based on the genetic foundation of human physiology, which hasn't changed much in the last 100,000 years. Genetically, says Sears, people aren't designed to eat pasta and other foods made from grain. Before humans invented agriculture and began growing grains, they hunted, fished, and gathered berries, nuts, roots, and leaves. According to Sears, his diet works because—in its emphasis on low-fat animal protein, fruit, and fiber-rich vegetables—it mimics the diet of our hunting and gathering ancestors. He cites a 1985 study describing neo-Paleolithic eating habits and claims that diet had the same protein-to-carbohydrate ratio as the diet he promotes. Sears has tested his diet on himself and his family, on people affected by heart disease, diabetes, and HIV, and also on elite athletes such as the Stanford University swim team. No control groups were used. He claims to have achieved excellent results overall and attributes eight gold medals won by Stanford swimmers at the 1992 Olympics to his diet.

The Method

How the Zone diet works

To enter the Zone, you have to figure out how many grams of protein your body needs on a daily basis. You spread out your protein allotment like a prescription drug, distributing it over three meals and two snacks and never allowing yourself to go more than five hours during the day without eating. You also need to stick to a good balance of carbs and protein. The ideal protein-to-carb ratio is.75, which means if you eat 7.5 grams of protein at one meal you would have 10 grams of carb to go along with it. To simplify the math, Sears converts everything into macronutrient "blocks": One protein block equals seven grams, one carbohydrate block equals nine grams, and one fat block equals one and a half grams. You eat the same number of blocks of protein, carb, and fat at each meal and snack, and this enables you to maintain the proper ratio. If, for example, you've determined that your body needs three blocks of protein at breakfast, then you would also eat three carb and three fat blocks. Sears lists typical macronutrient blocks to help you construct zone-favorable meals. For example, one block of protein works out to about an ounce of skinless chicken or turkey breast, two egg whites, an ounce of tuna, a quarter cup of low-fat cottage cheese, or a third of an ounce of protein powder. One block of carb could be a cup of cooked broccoli or zucchini, a tossed salad, a peach, half an orange or apple, or a quarter of a cantaloupe. One block of fat is equivalent to a teaspoon of olive oil and vinegar dressing, half a teaspoon of almond butter or natural peanut butter, one macadamia nut, three olives, or half a tablespoon of guacamole.

If the arithmetic of blocks drives you batty, you can try eyeballing portions using the palm of your hand as a gauge. The amount of protein you can hold in your hand is about equal to four blocks. To eyeball carbs, figure on about twice as much as the size of your protein portion. And add to that just a little fat—a little salad dressing or a few olives. Meanwhile, you should abide by one of Sears's central tenets: Try not to eat more than 500 calories per meal or 100 calories per snack, which adds up to no more than 1,700 calories daily.

Timing is important: For a person who eats breakfast at 7 a.m., the next meal should come no later than noon. A late afternoon snack will keep you in the Zone until dinner at 7 p.m., and a snack before bed will have you sleeping in the Zone until breakfast.

Sears recommends only low-fat protein; fiber-rich carbohydrates such as green beans, spinach, apples, and blueberries; and monounsaturated fats. Bad carbs, according to the author, include carrots, corn, peas, potatoes, sweet potatoes, bananas, raisins, prunes, papayas, all fruit juices (their fiber has been removed, and fiber slows down the speed at which food enters the bloodstream), most grains and breads, ice cream, honey, jelly, and granulated sugar.

What you'll notice

Sears doesn't say how much weight you'll lose or how long it will take. He does say you can expect some changes within five to seven days, which is how long it will supposedly take your body to make the hormonal adjustments necessary to catapult you into the Zone. Fatigue and listlessness, he vows, will disappear. You'll have more energy and focus, and you'll be calmer and more. After a while, he adds, you'll notice that you're healthier—less afflicted by colds, flus, and allergies. Sears says that if you have a chronic disease, treatment should become more manageable. Eventually you'll notice that you're eating enough to feel satisfied and yet you're still losing weight. Hunger-free weight loss, he assures you, will be virtually automatic.

Additional steps to take

Clearly, if you want to enter the Zone, you'll have do some calculations. First you determine your individual daily protein requirement, which depends on your weight, level of physical activity, and percentage of body fat. ears provides worksheets for figuring out your percentage of body fat; you'll also need a scale and a tape measure. Once you figure out your protein requirement, you can determine how much carb you should be eating.

What about vitamin and mineral supplements? Micronutrients, says the author, are not nearly as important as controlling the balance of macronutrients (protein, carb, and fat) in your diet. According to Sears, his diet supplies all the micronutrients you need except vitamin E. He recommends taking 200 IU of vitamin E daily, more than the minimum amount recommended by the government but not a megadose.

The Diet as Lifestyle

Staying the course

This diet is a total-health regimen, not solely a weight-loss program, and not surprisingly Sears has no advice about maintenance. His lifetime plan tightly controls "the balance of macronutrients" at "every meal, every snack, every day." Sears allows occasional indulgence in a carb-rich dessert as long some protein accompanies it. If you remain in the Zone, says Sears, you shouldn't have trouble with bingeing because his diet eliminates the sugar cravings that he claims drive you to binge in the first place. But if you do crave sweets, he suggests, you should look at what you ate at your last meal. Chances are you consumed too many carbs. To prevent this from happening again, he advises you to adjust your carb intake so that it more closely approximates the ideal ratio of one block of protein to one block of carb.

When you're traveling or at parties, Sears says comfortingly, you're out of the Zone just briefly, "only one meal away from reentering." He compares occasional dietary lapses to falling off a bike, advising you to "get back up and continue your journey."

Getting into gear

Sears encourages exercise and sees it as a vital part of any health program. When you've earned your passport to the Zone, he says, the benefits of exercise are enhanced. Aerobic exercise helps you burn excess body fat for energy. To get the real "sweat benefits" (improved weight control, cardiovascular fitness and strength), you need to devote a considerable amount of time to aerobic activity, Sears advises: six hours of walking a week or three hours of jogging. Higher-intensity aerobic exercise reduces levels of insulin and increases levels of glucagon, claims Sears, so your body ends up with a favorable ratio of good to bad eicosanoids and therefore releases more stored body fat to be used as fuel. He goes on to say that good eicosanoids dilate your blood vessels, increasing oxygen flow to the muscles and keeping you in a fat-burning mode for longer. High-intensity anaerobic exercise such as weight lifting is also beneficial, Sears maintains: It releases human growth hormone, which helps burn fat and build muscle.

To benefit most from any exercise, says Sears, you need to be in the Zone before, during, and after working out. He advises eating a Zone-favorable snack 30 minutes before exercise and again after exercising to help your body burn stored fat faster.

Evaluating the Diet

Cautions and concerns

While Sears's high-protein diet might work for some people trying to shed weight, the physiology behind his complex theory of good and bad eicosanoids has no scientific basis. It's true that eicosanoids play a role in blood clotting and the immune system, but they do not control "every cell, every organ, every system," as the author maintains. Nor is there evidence that eicosanoids are synthesized by this diet or any other. Any weight loss on Sears's plan comes from a drop in calories, not a hormonal sea change. The diet weighs in at about 1,000 to 1,700 calories daily.

Sears claims that 75 % of the population would have a hard time on a high-carb diet because elevated insulin levels cause them to accumulate body fat. This is putting the cart before the horse. Elevated insulin levels do not result in excess weight; rather, excess weight often results in the elevated insulin levels associated with a condition called insulin resistance. In fact, there is no reason to pin obesity on a diet rich in carbohydrate, unless that diet is also rich in calories. What about Sears's argument that humans are not genetically designed to eat pasta and other foods made from grain? Consider this: The Japanese eat a high-carb rice-based diet, and southern Mediterranean peoples eat a diet centered on pasta and olive oil. Both populations number among those with the longest life expectancy in the world.

One researcher actually undertook a study comparing a Zone-type, moderately-low-carb diet with a low-fat high-carb diet of equivalent calories. The results? Both groups lost the same amount of weight. So much for intricate theories about "good" and "bad" hormones regulating weight loss. When it comes to shedding pounds, it's simple: Calories count.

This diet discourages the consumption of whole-grain breads and cereals, which could result in constipation (from lack of fiber) and dehydration (carbs help your body store water). Simultaneously, the plan promotes heavy protein consumption, which can tax the liver and kidneys especially in people with preexisting disease—such as hepatitis—in those organs.

Quick fix or lasting results?

Sears makes no claims that you'll lose weight quickly on this diet, but he does say it will make a permanent change. If you do manage to stay on this low-cal plan you'll probably shed pounds. Keep in mind, however, that to keep your passport to the Zone, you'll have to eat twice the amount of protein that you would on a standard diet, and that could prove challenging in the long run.

Flexible or rigid?

You're allowed a wide variety of foods—indeed, nothing is absolutely forbidden. But the Zone's ideal carb-to-protein ratio might be difficult to enforce at every meal and for every snack. You also have to stick religiously to such rules as never going more than five hours without eating during the day.

Stumbling blocks

Despite Sears's proclamation—"once you've mastered the language of eicosanoids…your confusion about nutrition will simply evaporate"— some readers are likely to find his theories impenetrable. There's certainly no shortage of jargon within the pages of his book. Dieters considering this approach may also balk at the prospect of calculating the correct amount of protein, carb, and fat to be eaten throughout the day. Those who skip the theory and the numbers and simply try to follow the spirit of the diet may encounter another stumbling block: all that protein. If your body type mandates that you eat three "blocks" of protein for breakfast, you'd have to eat six egg whites (Sears discourages consumption of whole eggs), or three egg whites plus one and half ounces of lean Canadian bacon, or some other equivalent. On top of that, of course, you'd have to remember to consume the equivalent blocks of carb. When Sears conducted his own pilot study, he simply gave participants a prototype food bar with the correct ratio of macronutrients for breakfast.

Is it for you?

To follow the Zone approach, you have to be willing to think of food in a whole different way—not as a pleasure so much as a medicinal prescription. You also have to be rigorous about following a plan, constructing Zone-favorable meals with just the right ratio of ingredients. You'll be cutting back on foods that might be favorites as well, such as pastas. On the other hand, Sears does recommend a realtively plentiful pantry of healthy foods, including lean cuts of chicken and fish, abundant fruits and vegetables, healthy monounsaturated fats such as olive and canola oil, and oatmeal, if not pasta.

Don't follow this diet if you're pregnant, or if you have liver disease, kidney disease, or osteoporosis (the more protein you eat, the more calcium you excrete). Those with insulin-related disorders should check with the doctor before going on this diet because, contrary to common belief and Sears's claims, protein can stimulate insulin secretion, and there's protein in abundance on this plan.

Resources

Pick up a copy of *The Zone* (Harper Collins, l995) in your local bookstore, which may also carry other books by Sears: *Zone Perfect Meals in Minutes, The Anti-Aging Zone, Mastering the Zone: The Next Step in Achieving Superhealth and Permanent Fat Loss, A Week in the Zone*, and *The Soy Zone*. For additional information on this plan, visit the author's website at www.drsears.com.

Weight Goals

WEIGHT GOALS			
WOMEN			
Height	Small Frame	Medium Frame	Large Frame
4'10"	102-111 lbs.	109-121 lbs.	118-131 lbs.
4'11"	103-113	111-123	120-134
5'0"	104-115	113-126	122-137
5'1"	106-118	115-129	125-140
5'2"	108-121	118-132	128-143
5'3"	111-124	121-135	131-147
5'4"	114-127	124-138	134-151
5'5"	117-130	127-141	137-155
5'6"	120-133	130-144	140-159
5'7"	123-136	133-147	143-163
5'8"	126-139	136-150	146-167
5'9"	129-142	139-153	149-170
5'10"	132-145	142-156	152-173
5'11"	135-148	145-159	155-176
6'0"	138-151	148-162	158-179
MEN			
5'2"	128-134 lbs.	131-141 lbs.	138-150 lbs.
5'3"	130-136	133-143	140-153
5'4"	132-138	135-145	142-156
5'5"	134-140	137-148	144-160
5'6"	136-142	139-151	146-164
5'7"	138-145	142-154	149-168
5'8"	140-148	145-157	152-172
5'9"	142-151	148-160	155-176
5'10"	144-154	151-163	158-180
5'11"	146-157	154-166	161-184
6'0"	149-160	157-170	164-188
6'1"	152-164	160-174	168-192
6'2"	155-168	164-178	172-197
6'3"	158-172	167-182	176-202
6'4"	162-176	171-187	181-207

To determine your frame, use this trick: Encircle your wrist with your thumb and middle finger; if they overlap, you most likely have a small frame; if they touch, you're medium frame; if they don't touch, you have a large frame.

Food Content Guide

	Calories (kcal)	Protein (gm)
BEANS (LEGUMES) AND BEAN PRODUCTS		
Kidney beans, all types, boiled, without salt 1 cup	224.79	15.35
Peas, split, cooked, boiled, without salt 1 cup	231.28	16.35
Peanuts, all types, dry-roasted, with salt 1 oz.	165.85	6.71
Peanut butter, smooth style, with salt 2 tablespoons	189.76	8.07
Tofu, raw, regular 1 cup (1/2" cubes)	188.48	20.04
BEVERAGES		
Beer, regular 1 can (12 fl. oz.)	145.96	1.07
Beer, light 1 can (12 fl. oz.)	99.12	0.71
Wine, red 1 wine glass (3.5 fl. oz.)	74.16	0.21
Wine, rosé 1 wine glass (3.5 fl. oz.)	73.13	0.21
Wine, white 1 wine glass (3.5 fl. oz.)	70.04	0.1
Cola 1 can (16 fl. oz.)	201.72	0
Cola, diet, with aspartame 1 can (16 fl. oz.)	4.74	0.47
Ginger ale 1 can (16 fl. oz.)	165.92	0
Coffee, brewed, prep with tap water 1 cup (8 fl. oz.)	3.58	0.18
Tea, brewed, prep with tap water 1 cup (8 fl. oz.)	2.37	0
Tea, herb, chamomile, brewed	2.37	0

Carbohydrates (gm)	Fiber (gm)	Fat (gm)	Fat Saturated (gm)	Cholesterol (mg)
40.37	11.33	0.89	0.13	0
41.38	16.27	0.76	0.11	0
6.1	2.27	14.08	1.95	0
6.17	1.89	16.33	3.31	0
4.66	2.98	11.85	1.71	0
13.17	0.71	0	0	0
4.6	0	0	0	0
1.75	0	0	0	0
1.44	0	0	0	0
0.82	0	0	0	0
51.17	0	0	0	0
0.47	0	0	0	0
42.46	0	0	0	0
0.72	0	0	0	0
0.71	0	0	0	0
0.47	0	0	0	0

DAIRY PRODUCTS	Calories (kcal)	Protein (gm)
Butter, without salt 1 tablespoon	101.81	0.12
Blue cheese 1 oz.	100.09	6.07
Cheddar cheese 1 oz.	114.13	7.1
Cottage cheese, 1% fat 1 cup (not packed)	163.62	28
Cream cheese 1 tablespoon	1.09	0.39
Feta cheese 1 oz.	74.72	4.03
Mozzarella cheese, whole milk 1 oz.	79.77	5.51
Mozzarella cheese, part skim milk 1 oz.	72.08	6.88
Parmesan cheese, grated 1 tablespoon	22.79	2.08
Ricotta cheese, whole milk 1/2 cup	215.68	13.96
Ricotta cheese, part skim milk 1/2 cup	171.19	14.12
Swiss cheese 1 cup, diced	496.01	37.53
Egg, whole, raw, fresh 1 extra large	86.42	7.24
Egg, white, raw, fresh 1 large egg white	16.7	3.51
Egg, yolk, raw, fresh 1 large egg yolk	59.43	2.78
Milk, low-fat, 2% fat, with vit A 1 cup	121.2	8.13
Milk, fat-free (skim), with vit A 1 cup	85.53	8.35
Cream, light whipping 1 cup fluid (yields 2 cups whipped)	698.88	5.19
Cream, sour, cultured 1 tablespoon	25.71	0.38

Carbohydrates (gm)	Fiber (gm)	Fat (gm)	Fat Saturated (gm)	Cholesterol (mg)
0.01	0	11.52	7.17	31.08
0.66	0	8.15	5.29	21.32
0.36	0	9.40	5.98	29.74
6.15	0	2.31	1.46	9.94
0	5.06	3.19	15.9	
1.16	0	6.03	4.24	25.23
0.63	0	6.12	3.73	22.23
0.79	0	4.51	2.87	16.39
0.19	0	1.5	0.95	3.94
3.77	0	16.1	10.29	62.74
6.37	0	9.81	6.11	38.19
4.46	0	36.23	23.47	121.04
0.71	0	5.81	1.8	246.5
0.34	0	0	0	0
0.3	0	5.12	1.59	212.65
11.71	0	4.68	2.92	18.3
11.88	0	0.44	0.29	4.41
7.07	0	73.87	46.22	265.29
0.51	0	2.52	1.57	5.33

	Calories (kcal)	Protein (gm)
Ice cream, chocolate 1/2 cup (4 fl. oz.)	142.56	2.51
Ice cream, strawberry 1/2 cup (4 fl. oz.)	126.72	2.11
Ice cream, vanilla 1/2 cup (4 fl. oz.)	132.66	2.31
Yogurt, plain, whole milk 1 cup (8 fl. oz.)	150.48	8.5
Yogurt, plain, low-fat 1 cup (8 fl. oz.)	155.05	12.86
Yogurt, plain, fat-free (skim) milk 1 cup (8 fl. oz.)	136.64	14.04

FATS AND OILS

	Calories (kcal)	Protein (gm)
Margarine, reg, hard, corn (hydrogenated) 1 teaspoon	33.78	0.04
Margarine, soft, corn (hydrogenated and reg) 1 teaspoon	33.67	0.04
Canola oil 1 tablespoon	123.76	0
Corn, salad or cooking oil 1 tablespoon	120.22	0
Olive, salad or cooking oil 1 tablespoon	119.34	0
Sesame, salad or cooking oil 1 tablespoon	120.22	0

FRUITS AND FRUITS JUICES

	Calories (kcal)	Protein (gm)
Apples, raw, with skin 1 cup, quartered or chopped	73.75	0.24
Apple juice, canned or bottled, unsweetened, with vit C 1 cup	116.56	0.15
Apricots, raw 1 cup, halves	74.4	2.17
Avocados, raw 1 fruit, without skin and pit	306.21	3.65

Carbohydrates (gm)	Fiber (gm)	Fat (gm)	Fat Saturated (gm)	Cholesterol (mg)
18.61	0.79	7.26	4.49	22.44
18.22	0.2	5.54	3.43	19.14
15.58	0	7.26	4.48	29.04
11.42	0	7.96	5.14	31.12
17.25	0	3.8	2.45	14.9
18.82	0	0.44	0.28	4.41
0.04	0	3.78	0.62	0
0.02	0	3.78	0.66	0
0	0	14	.99	0
0	0	13.6	1.73	0
0	0	13.5	1.82	0
0	0	13.6	1.93	0
19.06	3.38	0.45	0.07	0
28.97	0.25	0.27	0.05	0
17.24	3.72	0.6	0.04	0
11.95	8.48	29.98	2.28	0

	Calories (kcal)	Protein (gm)
Bananas, raw 1 cup, sliced	138	1.55
Blueberries, raw 1 pint	225.12	2.69
Cherries, sweet, raw 1 cup, with pits	84.24	1.4
Grapefruit, raw, pink and red and white 1 cup sections, with juice	73.6	1.45
Grapefruit juice, canned, unsweetened 1 cup	93.86	1.28
Grapes, American type (slip skin), raw 1 cup	57.96	0.58
Grape juice, canned or bottled, unsweetened, without vit C 1 cup	154.33	1.42
Lemon juice 1 fl. oz.	7.63	0.12
Mangos, raw 1 fruit, without refuse	134.55	1.06
Melons, cantaloupe, raw 1 cup, balls	61.95	1.56
Melons, honeydew, raw 1 cup, diced (approx. 20 pieces per cup)	59.5	0.78
Nectarines, raw 1 fruit (2 1/2" dia)	66.64	1.28
Oranges, raw, Florida 1 fruit (2 5/8" dia)	64.86	0.99
Orange juice, raw 1 cup	111.6	1.74
Tangerines (mandarin oranges), canned, juice pk 1 cup	92.13	1.54
Peaches, raw 1 large (2 3/4" dia; approx. 2 1/2 per lb.)	67.51	1.1
Pears, raw 1 medium (approx. 2 1/2 per lb.)	97.94	0.65
Pineapple, raw 1 cup, diced	75.97	0.6
Plums, raw 1 fruit (2 1/8" dia)	36.3	0.52
Prunes, dried, uncooked 1 fruit	20.08	0.22

Carbohydrates (gm)	Fiber (gm)	Fat (gm)	Fat Saturated (gm)	Cholesterol (mg)
35.15	3.6	0.72	0.28	0
56.8	10.85	1.53	0.13	0
19.36	2.69	1.12	0.25	0
18.58	2.53	0.23	0.03	0
22.13	0.25	0.25	0.03	0
15.78	0.92	0.32	0.1	0
37.85	0.25	0.2	0.06	0
2.63	0.12	0	0	0
35.19	3.73	0.56	0.14	0
14.8	1.42	0.5	0.13	0
15.61	1.02	0.17	0.04	0
16.02	2.18	0.63	0.07	0
16.27	3.38	0.3	0.04	0
25.79	0.5	0.5	0.06	0
23.83	1.74	0.07	0.01	0
17.43	3.14	0.14	0.02	0
25.08	3.98	0.66	0.04	0
19.2	1.86	0.67	0.05	0
8.59	0.99	0.41	0.03	0
5.27	0.6	0.04	0	0

	Calories (kcal)	Protein (gm)
Raisins, seedless 1 cup, packed	495	5.31
Raspberries, raw 1 cup	60.27	1.12
Strawberries, raw 1 cup, halves	45.6	0.93

GRAIN PRODUCTS

	Calories (kcal)	Protein (gm)
Bagels, plain, enriched, with calcium propionate (including onion, poppy, sesame) 1 bagel (3" dia)	156.75	5.99
Bread crumbs, dry, grated, plain 1 cup	426.6	13.5
Dinner rolls, wheat 1 roll (1 oz.)	77.4	2.44
English muffins, plain, enriched, with calcium propionate (including sourdough) 1 muffin	133.95	4.39
Hamburger or hotdog, plain rolls 1 roll	122.98	3.66
Hard (including Kaiser) rolls 1 roll (3 1/2" dia)	167.01	5.65
Mixed-grain (including whole-grain, 7-grain) bread 1 large slice	80	3.2
Pita, white, enriched bread 1 large (6 1/2" dia)	165	5.46
Rye bread 1 slice	82.88	2.72
Wheat (including wheat berry) bread 1 slice	65	2.28
White bread, commercially prep 1 slice	40	1
Taco shells, baked 1 large (6 1/2" dia	98.28	1.51
Tortillas, ready-to-bake or –fry, corn 1 medium (approx. 6" dia)	1.48	12.12
Tortillas, ready-to-bake or –fry, flour 1 medium (approx. 6" dia)	2.78	17.79
Saltine crackers (including oyster, soda, soup) 1 cup, oyster crackers	195.3	4.14

Carbohydrates (gm)	Fiber (gm)	Fat (gm)	Fat Saturated (gm)	Cholesterol (mg)
130.56	6.6	0.76	0.25	0
14.23	8.36	0.68	0.02	0
10.67	3.5	0.56	0.03	0
30.44	1.31	0.91	0.13	0
78.3	2.59	5.83	1.36	0
13.04	1.07	1.79	0.43	0
26.22	1.54	1.03	0.15	0
21.63	1.16	2.19	0.51	0
30.04	1.31	2.45	0.35	0
14.85	2.05	1.22	0.6	0
33.42	1.32	0.72	0.1	0
15.46	1.86	1.06	0.2	0
11.8	1.08	1.03	0.22	0
7	0	0.5	0.1	0
13.1	1.58	4.75	0.7	0
1.35	45.5	0.65	0.09	0
1.06	40	2.27	0.35	0
32.8	1.35	5.31	0.95	0

	Calories (kcal)	Protein (gm)
Wheat crackers, regular 1 cracker	18.92	0.34
Wheat flour, whole-grain 1 cup	406.8	16.44
Wheat flour, white, all-purpose, enriched 1 cup	455	12.91
Couscous, cooked 1 cup	175.84	5.95
Oat bran, cooked 1 cup	87.6	7.03
Oats, instant, fortified, plain, prep with water 1 cup	138.06	5.85
Rice, brown, long-grain, cooked 1 cup	216.45	5.03
Rice, brown, medium-grain, cooked 1 cup	218.4	4.52
Rice, white, long-grain, reg, cooked, enriched, with salt 1 cup	205.4	4.25
Wheat germ, toasted, plain 1 cup	43.66	32.88
Wild rice, cooked 1 cup	165.64	6.54
Macaroni, cooked, enriched 1 cup elbow shaped	197.4	6.68
Noodles, egg, cooked, enriched 1 cup	212.8	7.6
Spaghetti, cooked, enriched, without salt 1 cup	197.4	6.68

CONDIMENTS

Catsup 1 tablespoon	15.6	0.23
Garlic, raw 1 teaspoon	4.17	0.18
Pickles, cucumber, dill 1 cup (about 23 slices)	27.9	0.96
Pickles, cucumber, sweet 1 cup, sliced	198.9	0.63
Pickle relish, sweet 1 tablespoon	19.5	0.06

Carbohydrates (gm)	Fiber (gm)	Fat (gm)	Fat Saturated (gm)	Cholesterol (mg)
2.6	0.18	0.82	0.15	0
87.08	14.64	2.24	0.39	0
95.39	3.38	1.23	0.19	0
36.46	2.2	0.84	0.15	0
25.05	5.69	1.88	0.36	0
23.87	3.98	2.34	0.42	0
44.77	3.51	1.76	0.35	0
45.84	3.51	1.62	0.32	0
44.1	0.63	0.44	0.12	0
56.05	14.58	12.09	2.07	0
35	2.95	0.56	0.08	0
39.68	1.82	0.94	0.13	0
39.74	1.76	2.35	0.5	5.8
39.68	2.38	0.94	0.13	0
4.09	0.2	0.05	0.01	0
0.93	0.06	0.01	0	0
6.4	1.86	0.29	0.07	0
54.08	1.87	0.44	0.11	0
5.26	0.17	0.07	0.01	0

	Calories (kcal)	Protein (gm)
MEAT: BEEF		
Chuck, arm pot roast, lean and fat, 1/4" fat, braised 3 oz.	282.2	23.32
Shortribs, lean and fat, choice, braised 3 oz.	400.35	18.33
Bottom round, lean and fat, 1/4" fat all grades, braised 3 oz.	233.75	24.36
Eye of round, lean and fat, 1/4" fat, all roasted 3 oz.	194.65	22.77
Tenderloin, lean and fat, 1/4" fat, broiled 3 oz.	247.35	21.47
Ground, extra lean, broiled, well done	225.25	24.29
Ground, lean, broiled, well done	238	23.97
Ground, regular, broiled, well done	248.2	23.12
LAMB		
Domestic, leg, whole (shk and sirl), lean, 1/4" fat, choice, roasted. 3 oz.	162.35	24.06
Domestic, loin, lean and fat, 1/4" fat, choice, roasted 3 oz.	262.65	19.17
Domestic, cubed for stew, leg and shoulder), lean, 1/4" fat, braised. 3 OZ.	189.55	28.64
VEAL		
Leg, lean, roasted 3 oz.	127.5	23.86
Loin, lean, roasted 3 oz.	148.75	22.37
Rib, lean, roasted 3 oz.	150.45	21.9
PORK		
Fresh, (ham), whole, lean, roasted 3 oz.	179.35	25

Carbohydrates (gm)	Fiber (gm)	Fat (gm)	Fat Saturated (gm)	Cholesterol (mg)
0	0	20.24	7.97	84.15
0	0	35.68	15.13	79.9
0	0	14.37	5.41	81.6
0	0	10.84	4.23	61.2
0	0	17.22	6.76	73.1
0	0	13.43	5.28	84.15
0	0	14.99	5.89	85.85
0	0	16.54	6.50	85.85
0	0	6.58	2.35	75.65
0	0	20.05	8.7	80.75
0	0	7.48	2.68	91.8
0	0	2.88	1.04	87.55
0	0	5.9	2.19	90.1
0	0	6.32	1.77	97.75
0	0	8.02	2.81	79.9

	Calories (kcal)	Protein (gm)
Fresh, loin, whole, lean, roasted 3 oz.	177.65	24.33
Fresh , center loin (chops), bone-in, lean, broiled 3 oz.	171.7	25.66
Fresh, sirloin (roasts), bone-in, lean, roasted 3 oz.	183.6	24.49
Fresh, spareribs, lean and fat, braised 3 oz.	337.45	24.7
Cured, bacon, broiled, pan-fried or roasted 3 medium slices, after cooking	109.44	5.79
Cured, Canadian-style bacon, grilled 2 slices (6 per 6 oz. pkg.)	86.03	11.27
Cured, ham, boneless, extra lean (approx. 5% fat), roasted 3 oz.	12.25	17.79
Cured, ham, whole, lean, roasted 3 oz.	133.45	21.29
POULTRY		
Chicken, light meat, meat and skin, roasted 1/2 chicken, one removed	293.04	38.31
Chicken, dark meat, meat and skin, roasted 1/2 chicken, bone removed	422.51	43.37
Chicken, light meat, meat only, fried 1 cup	268.8	45.95
Chicken, light meat, meat only, roasted 1 cup, chopped or diced	242.2	43.27
Chicken, dark meat, meat only, fried 1 cup	334.6	40.59
Chicken, dark meat, meat only, roasted 1 cup, chopped or diced	287	38.32
Cornish game hens, meat only, roasted 1/2 bird	147.4	25.63
Duck, domesticated, meat only, roasted 1 cup, chopped or diced	281.4	32.87
Turkey, all classes, light meat, cooked, roasted 1 cup, chopped or diced	219.8	41.86
Turkey, all classes, dark meat, cooked, roasted 1 cup, chopped or diced	261.8	39.1

Carbohydrates (gm)	Fiber (gm)	Fat (gm)	Fat Saturated (gm)	Cholesterol (mg)
0	0	8.19	2.98	68.85
0	0	6.86	2.51	69.7
0	0	8.75	3.08	73.1
0	0	25.76	9.45	102.85
0.11	0	9.36	3.31	16.15
0.63	0	3.92	1.32	26.97
1.28	0	4.7	1.54	45.0
0	0	4.68	1.56	46.75
0	0	14.32	4.03	110.88
0	0	26.35	7.3	151.97
0.59	0	7.76	2.13	126
0	0	6.31	1.78	119
3.63	0	16.27	4.37	134.4
0	0	13.62	3.72	130.2
0	0	4.26	1.09	116.6
0	0	15.68	5.84	124.6
0	0	4.51	1.44	96.6
0	0	10.11	3.39	119

	Calories (kcal)	Protein (gm)
LUNCHEON MEAT		
Bologna, beef 1 slice (4" dia x 1/8" thick)	71.76	2.81
Frankfurter, beef 1 frankfurter (5" long x 3/4" dia; 10 per pound)	141.75	5.4
Ham, sliced, extra lean, (approx. 5% fat) 1 slice (6 1/4" x 4" x 1/16")	37.14	5.49
Salami, beef and pork 1 slice (4" dia x 1/8" thick; 10 per 8 oz. package)	57.5	3.2
Turkey breast meat 1 slice (3 1/2" square; 8 per 6 oz. package)	23.1	4.73
Turkey roll, light meat 2 slices	83.35	10.6
NUTS, SEEDS, AND RELATED PRODUCTS		
Almonds, dry roasted, unblanched, without salt 1 cup whole kernels	810.06	22.54
Cashew nuts, dry roasted, without salt 1 cup, halves and whole	786.38	20.97
Coconut meat, raw 1 cup, shredded	283.2	2.66
Coconut meat, dried (desiccated), not sweetened 1 oz.	187.11	1.95
Filberts or hazelnuts, dry roasted, unblanched, without salt 1 oz.	187.68	2.84
Macadamia nuts, dried 1 oz. (11 whole kernels)	199.02	2.35
Olives, ripe, canned (small-extra large) 1 large	5.06	0.04
Pecans, dry roasted, without salt 1 oz.	186.83	2.26
Pistachio nuts, dry roasted, without salt 1 cup	775.68	19.11
Walnuts, black, dried 1 cup, chopped	758.75	30.44

Carbohydrates (gm)	Fiber (gm)	Fat (gm)	Fat Saturated (gm)	Cholesterol (mg)
0.18	0	6.56	2.78	13.34
0.81	0	12.83	5.42	27.45
0.27	0	1.41	0.46	13.32
0.52	0	4.63	1.86	14.95
0	0	0.33	0.1	8.61
0.3	0	4.09	1.15	24.38
33.35	18.91	71.21	6.75	0
44.79	4.11	63.5	12.55	0
12.18	7.2	26.79	23.76	0
6.92	4.62	18.29	16.22	0
5.07	2.04	18.8	1.38	0
3.89	2.64	20.9	3.13	0
0.28	0.14	0.47	0.06	0
6.33	2.64	18.31	1.47	0
35.24	13.82	67.61	8.56	0
15.13	6.25	70.73	4.54	0

SEAFOOD	Calories (kcal)	Protein (gm)
Bass, freshwater, mixed species, cooked, dry heat 3 oz.	124.1	20.55
Bass, striped, cooked, dry heat 3 oz.	105.4	19.32
Carp, cooked, dry heat 3 oz.	137.7	19.43
Caviar, black and red, granular 1 tablespoon	40.32	3.94
Cod, Atlantic, cooked, dry heat 3 oz.	89.25	19.41
Flat fish (flounder and sole species), cooked, dry heat 3 oz.	99.45	20.54
Haddock, cooked, dry heat 3 oz.	95.2	20.6
Halibut, Atlantic and Pacific, cooked, dry heat 3 oz.	119	22.69
Herring, Atlantic, pickled 1 oz., boneless	74.28	4.02
Mackerel, Atlantic, cooked, dry heat 3 oz.	222.7	20.27
Monkfish, cooked, dry heat 3 oz.	82.45	15.78
Perch, mixed species, cooked, dry heat 3 oz.	99.45	21.13
Roe, mixed species, cooked, dry heat 1 oz.	57.83	8.11
Roughy, orange, cooked, dry heat 3 oz.	75.65	16.02
Salmon, chinook, smoked (lox), reg 3 oz.	99.45	15.54
Salmon, pink, cooked, dry heat 3 oz.	126.65	21.73
Sardine, Atlantic, canned in oil, drained solids with bone 1 oz.	58.97	6.98
Sea bass, mixed species, cooked, dry heat 3 oz.	105.4	20.09
Snapper, mixed species, cooked, dry heat 3 oz.	108.8	22.36

Carbohydrates (gm)	Fiber (gm)	Fat (gm)	Fat Saturated (gm)	Cholesterol (mg)
0	0	4.02	0.85	73.95
0	0	2.54	0.55	87.55
0	0	6.09	1.18	71.4
0.64	0	2.86	0.65	94.08
0	0	0.73	0.14	46.75
0	0	1.3	0.31	57.8
0	0	0.79	0.14	62.9
0	0	2.5	0.35	34.85
2.73	0	5.1	0.68	3.69
0	0	15.14	3.55	63.75
0	0	1.66	0	27.2
0	0	1	0.2	97.75
0.54	0	2.33	0.53	135.8
0	0	0.77	0.02	22.1
0	0	3.67	0.79	19.55
0	0	3.76	0.61	56.95
0	0	3.25	0.43	40.26
0	0	2.18	0.56	45.05
0	0	1.46	0.31	39.95

	Calories (kcal)	Protein (gm)
Swordfish, cooked, dry heat 3 oz.	131.75	21.58
Trout, rainbow, wild, cooked, dry heat 3 oz.	127.5	19.48
Tuna, fresh, bluefin, cooked, dry heat 3 oz.	156.4	25.42
Tuna, white, canned in oil, drained solids 3 oz.	158.1	22.55
Tuna, white, canned in water, drained solids 3 oz.	108.8	20.08
Clam, mixed species, cooked, moist heat 20 small	281.2	48.55
Crab, Alaska king, cooked, moist heat 1 leg	29.98	25.93
Lobster, northern, cooked, moist heat 3 oz.	83.3	17.43
Mussel, blue, cooked, moist heat 3 oz.	146.2	20.23
Oyster, eastern, raw 6 medium	57.12	5.92
Scallop, mixed species, cooked, breaded and fried 2 large	138.55	16.07
Shrimp, mixed species, cooked, moist heat 4 large	21.78	4.6

VEGETABLES AND VEGETABLE JUICES

	Calories (kcal)	Protein (gm)
Artichokes (globe or French), cooked, boiled, drained, without salt. 1 medium	60	4.18
Asparagus, raw 1 small spear (5" long or less)	2.76	0.27
Beans, snap, green, cooked, boiled, drained, without salt 1 cup	43.75	2.36
Broccoli, raw 1 cup, flowerets	19.88	2.12
Brussels sprouts, cooked, boiled, drained, without salt 1/2 cup	30.42	1.99
Cabbage, raw 1 cup, shredded	17.5	1.01

Carbohydrates (gm)	Fiber (gm)	Fat (gm)	Fat Saturated (gm)	Cholesterol (mg)
0	0	4.37	1.2	42.5
0	0	4.95	1.38	58.65
0	0	5.34	1.37	41.65
0	0	6.87	1.4	26.35
0	0	2.53	0.67	35.7
9.75	0	3.71	0.36	127.3
0	0	2.06	0.18	71.02
1.09	0	0.5	0.09	61.2
6.28	0	3.81	0.72	47.6
3.28	0	2.07	0.65	44.52
8.42	0	3.91	0.87	85
0	0	0.24	0.06	42.9
13.42	6.48	0.19	0.04	0
0.54	0.25	0.02	0.01	0
9.86	4	0.35	0.08	0
3.72	2.13	0.25	0.04	0
6.76	2.03	0.4	0.08	0
3.8	1.61	0.19	0.02	0

	Calories (kcal)	Protein (gm)
Cabbage, red, raw 1 cup, shredded	18.9	0.97
Carrots, raw 1 cup, grated	47.3	1.13
Cauliflower, raw 1 cup	25	1.98
Celery, raw 1 cup, diced	19.2	0.9
Corn, sweet, yellow, cooked, boiled, drained, without salt 1 baby ear	8.64	0.27
Cucumber, with peel, raw 1/2 cup, slices	6.76	0.36
Lettuce, cos or romaine, raw 1/2 cup, shredded	4.48	0.45
Lettuce, iceberg (including crisphead types), raw 1 cup, shredded or chopped	6.6	0.56
Mushrooms, raw 1 cup, whole	24	2.01
Mushrooms, shiitake, dried 1 mushroom	10.66	0.34
Onions, raw 1 cup, chopped	60.8	1.86
Onions, spring (including tops and bulb), raw 1 tablespoon, chopped	1.92	0.11
Parsley, raw 1 cup	21.6	1.78
Peas, green, cooked, boiled, drained, without salt 1 cup	134.4	8.58
Peppers, sweet, green, raw 1 cup, chopped	40.23	1.33
Potatoes, baked, flesh, without salt 1 potato (2 1/3" x 4 3/4")	145.08	3.06
Spinach, cooked, boiled, drained, without salt 1 cup	41.4	5.35
Squash, summer, zucchini, including skin, raw 1 cup, sliced	15.82	1.31
Sweet potato, cooked, baking in skin, without salt 1 large	185.4	3.1
Tomatoes, red, ripe, raw, year round average 1 cup, chopped or sliced	37.8	1.53

Carbohydrates (gm)	Fiber (gm)	Fat (gm)	Fat Saturated (gm)	Cholesterol (mg)
4.28	1.4	0.18	0.02	0
11.15	3.3	0.21	0.03	0
5.2	2.5	0.21	0.03	0
4.38	2.04	0.17	0.04	0
2.01	0.22	0.1	0.02	0
1.44	0.42	0.07	0.02	0
0.66	0.48	0.06	0.01	0
1.15	0.77	0.1	0.01	0
4.46	1.15	0.4	0.05	0
2.71	0.41	0.04	0.01	0
13.81	2.88	0.26	0.04	0
0.44	0.16	0.01	0	0
3.8	1.98	0.47	0.08	0
25.02	8.8	0.35	0.06	0
9.58	2.68	0.28	0.04	0
33.63	2.34	0.16	0.04	0
6.75	4.32	0.47	0.08	0
3.28	1.36	0.16	0.03	0
43.69	5.4	0.2	0.04	0
8.35	1.98	0.59	0.08	0

Counting Calories

Here are 50 good food choices if you are counting calories.
See the main chart for more calorie counts.

Description	Calories	Description	Calories
Beverages		**Fruits**	
Grapefruit juice, unsweetened 1 cup	93.86	Tangerine 1 fruit	43.12
Orange juice 1 cup	111.6	Plum 1 fruit	36.3
Skim milk 1 cup	85.53	Raspberries 1 cup	60.27
Coffee 1 cup	3.58	Strawberries 1 cup	45.6
Tea 1 cup	2.37	Watermelon 1 cup	51
Red wine 1 glass	74.16	Fruit sorbet 1/2 cup	130
Milk, low-fat (2%) 1 cup	121.2		

Description	Calories	Description	Calories
Vegetables			
Broccoli, raw 1 cup	19.88	Eggplant, boiled 1 cup	27.72
Carrots, boiled 1/2 cup	35.1	Endive 1/2 cup, chopped	4.25
Cauliflower, raw 1 cup	25	Mushrooms, raw 1 cup	24
Cauliflower 1/2 cup	14.26	Spinach, boiled 1 cup	41.4
Celery 1 cup, diced	19.2	Zucchini, boiled 1 cup	37.91
Sweet yellow corn 1 ear	8.64	Tomatoes 1 cup	37.8
Cucumber, with peel, raw 1/2 cup	6.76	Salsa 2 tbsp.	6

Description	Calories	Description	Calories
Grains		**Dairy**	
Breadsticks, plain 1 small stick	20.6	Plain, fat-free yogurt 1 cup	136.64
Wheat bread 1 slice	65		
White bread 1 slice	40		
Tortilla, flour 1 medium	2.78		
Oat bran, cooked 1 cup	87.6		
Wild rice, cooked 1 cup	165.64		
Spaghetti, cooked 1 cup	197.4		
Popcorn, air popped, without butter or salt 1 cup	31		
Fish and Meat			
Monkfish, cooked, dry heat 3 oz.	82.45	Ham, sliced, extra lean 4 slices	148.56
Snapper, cooked, dry heat 3 oz.	108.8	Chicken, light meat, roasted 1 cup	242.2
Rainbow trout, cooked, dry heat 3 oz.	127.5	Lamb, leg, lean, roasted 3 oz.	162.35
Tuna, light, canned in water, drained 3 oz.	98.6	Pork chops, center loin, lean, broiled 3 oz.	171.7

Index